The Convergence of Science and Governance

The Convergence of Science and Governance

Research, Health Policy, and American States

DANIEL M. FOX

University of California Press

BERKELEY   LOS ANGELES   LONDON

University of California Press, one of the most distinguished
university presses in the United States, enriches lives around the world
by advancing scholarship in the humanities, social sciences, and natural
sciences. Its activities are supported by the UC Press Foundation and
by philanthropic contributions from individuals and institutions. For
more information, visit www.ucpress.edu.

University of California Press
Berkeley and Los Angeles, California

University of California Press, Ltd.
London, England

Library of Congress Cataloging-in-Publication Data

Fox, Daniel M.
   The convergence of science and governance : research, health policy,
and American states / Daniel M. Fox.
      p.   cm.
   Includes bibliographical references and index.
   ISBN 978-0-520-26238-6 (cloth : alk. paper)
   1. Medical policy—United States.   2. Pharmaceutical policy—
United States.   3. National Health Services—United States.   I. Title.
   [DNLM: 1. Insurance, pharmaceutical services—History—United
States.   2. Government programs—History—United States.
3. Health policy—History—United States.   4. Health services
research—History—United States.   5. History, 20th century—United
States.   6. History, 21st century—United States.   7. Politics—United
States.   W 265 AA1 F791c 2010]

RA395.A3F684   2010
362.1—dc22   2009019420

Manufactured in the United States of America

19 18 17 16 15 14 13 12 11 10
10 9 8 7 6 5 4 3 2 1

This book is printed on Cascades Enviro 100, a 100% post consumer
waste, recycled, de-inked fiber. FSC recycled certified and processed
chlorine free. It is acid free, Ecologo certified, and manufactured by
BioGas energy.

Contents

Preface: Converging Stories

This book tells related stories about health politics and policy in the United States during the past century. The story that frames the book is the recent convergence of science and governance in policy for covering pharmaceutical drugs in public programs in most American states. The other stories explain why and how this convergence occurred.

A story fundamental to convergence is how politics has influenced the questions, methods, and reception of research on health services during the past century. The politics of research is part of a larger political struggle over who will do what, to, for and with whom, using what resources, to prevent and treat disease and its consequences. Interest groups are central in politics. But health politics is also about competing ideas and values that become conflicting opinions about power and money—especially opinions about social justice, the accountability of health professionals, the uses of technology, and the missions, structure and management of health-care organizations. The burden of disease and disability, and how it changes over time, is a constant, though often understated, force in the politics of health.

Another essential story in this book is how officials of state government have used policy to protect, maintain, and improve the health of populations and the individuals who comprise them. Much of the health policy that states have made and implemented since the nineteenth century has been independent of the federal government. State policy has often responded to federal mandates and incentives. But states have also influenced federal policy.

The history of the politics of research on health services and of governance in the states made convergence possible. Events in the general economy and in state and national politics made it feasible. Particular policymakers in state government and their advisers made it happen.

Two related stories about these policymakers thread through the book. One is how they learned about the methods and came to appreciate the potential uses of research on health services. The other story is how they initiated, sustained, and defended the convergence of science and governance.

There are grounds for anxiety about the fragility of convergence, as well as for predicting that it will expand in scope. I also tell and assess these potential stories.

The stories in this book are grounded in my reading of archival and published primary sources and draw on an extensive secondary literature. But I also use my experience of helping to make and implement policy over four decades.

For most of my career, I compartmentalized my work in public affairs and research. During the 1960s I recognized that I was committed to both government work and scholarship. I observed, however, that many public officials are dismissive of intellectuals in government, and that many academics assume that public officials are their inferiors in conceptualizing and analyzing problems and potential solutions to them.

I separated my careers in order to achieve professional standing in each of them. I achieved separation by devising different voices for writing in each career; and named them the Narrator and the Bureaucrat in an essay published in 1985.[1] The Narrator wrote mainly for people who did research, health professionals, advanced students, and, when he could, for general readers. The Bureaucrat wrote for people who worked in the legislative and executive branches of federal, state, and local government.

The Narrator was "a relativist, an ironist, an existentialist"; an exemplary academic of his generation. He "believes that there is no past except what we create in the present and that most problems that now appear to be solved will, in time, most likely also appear to be trivial."

The Bureaucrat, in contrast, was "a technocrat, a moralist, a cynic." He was a technocrat because making policy requires immersion in esoteric details; a moralist because policymakers must assess value and make hard choices to allocate scarce resources; and a cynic because most people interpret the past and try to shape the present in ways that promote their ideology or self-interest. To be effective in politics, however, cynics must attend to their obligations. The Bureaucrat was, therefore, intensely loyal to his friends.

The Narrator and the Bureaucrat had some success for three decades. Academics did not condemn the Narrator's articles and books for having polemical purposes or for being autobiography disguised as history. The

Bureaucrat wrote a vast amount of ephemeral prose that helped to create, defend, and, at times, prevent particular policy.

The Narrator and the Bureaucrat began to collaborate in 1993 when the Narrator wrote the first four chapters of a book and the Bureaucrat wrote its conclusion.[2] For the first time, I used my experience in politics and policymaking as primary sources for scholarly writing. I had begun to invite readers to judge my experience as they would any other evidence.

I have used personal experience as a source, along with standard primary and secondary sources, in most subsequent articles and public talks. The Narrator and the Bureaucrat have also converged.

Acknowledgments

Colleagues in government and research since the 1960s participated in many of the events I describe. I owe a particular debt to members of the Reforming States Group (RSG). These policymakers from the United States, Canada, Australia, England, and Scotland have been central to the story of convergence that frames the book and essential to my being able to tell it. Similarly, members of the governance of the Drug Effectiveness Review Project (DERP) provided important information and suggestions about interpreting it.

Eight colleagues read the book in draft. Lynne Withey (University of California Press) encouraged me to "say straight out that this is a success story" and to emphasize that the "story is about state governments—and maybe that is one reason for success." Mark Gibson (Center for Evidence-Based Policy) helped me to describe and interpret events in which he participated and made helpful suggestions about style. Lee Greenfield (retired from the Minnesota House of Representatives and Hennepin County government) read the manuscript in the context of his personal experience of much of the history in this book. John McDonough (U.S. Senate, Committee on Health, Education, Labor and Pensions) assessed the book on the basis of his careers as a policymaker in state and federal government and as an author. Steven Lewis (Access Consulting) encouraged me to emphasize that the stories I tell exemplify my views about the general characteristics of effective health politics. David Rosner (Columbia University) recommended a strategy for calling readers' attention at the beginning of the book to the broader history that made the framing story possible. David also helped me to clarify the relationship between the history of social medicine and research on the effectiveness of health services. Howard Markel (University of Michigan) urged me to emphasize the history of research and of health politics that made convergence possible. Kathleen S. Andersen (Milbank Memorial Fund), who has also written about the history of the RSG, has long been an indispensable source of information and advice.

Other colleagues responded generously to my requests for assistance. Iain Chalmers (James Lind Library), Andrew Oxman (Norwegian Knowledge Center for the Health Services), Mark Helfand (Oregon Health and Sciences University), David Henry (Institute for Clinical Evaluative Sciences), and Peter Tugwell (University of Ottawa) helped me understand the history of the science of research synthesis, to which each of them has contributed. Edward D. Berkowitz (George Washington University), Nick Black (London School of Hygiene and Tropical Medicine), Bradford H. Gray (Urban Institute and the Milbank Memorial Fund), Kenneth Ludmerer (Washington University), and Gerald Oppenheimer (Brooklyn College, City University of New York) provided advice on other issues in the history of health politics and policy. Jessie Gruman (Center for the Advancement of Health) and Clarion E. Johnson Jr. (ExxonMobil) have informed my understanding of the problems of sustaining convergence. Eileen Cody (Washington State House of Representatives) and Bob Nakagawa (Ministry of Health, British Columbia), Pam Curtis and Alison Little (Center for Evidence-Based Policy), John Santa (formerly at the Center, now at Consumers Union), Gail Shearer (Consumers Union), James Thompson (Federation of State Medical Boards), and David Helms (Academy Health) provided timely information while I was writing.

The Milbank Memorial Fund has been associated with the stories I tell in this book since early in the twentieth century. I am grateful to Tony Milbank, chairman of its board, and Carmen Hooker Odom, my successor as its president, for encouragement, advice and friendship.

1. Why Convergence? Why Now?

This book describes and sets in context extraordinary recent events in policymaking for health in American states. Between 2001 and 2008, most states began to make policy as a result of which independent research informs decisions about coverage for pharmaceutical drugs for persons enrolled in Medicaid and the State Children's Health Insurance Program; and, in a growing number of states, for other health programs.[1] Spending for these programs totals billions of dollars each year. They pay for health care for almost a quarter of Americans.[2] Medicaid is, moreover, the largest payer for prenatal care, childbirth, and AIDS/HIV.

These events struck journalists, experts on health policy, and executives in the pharmaceutical industry as unusual because:

- Policymakers in the legislative and executive branches of state government made policy that facilitated applying findings derived from methods of research in which the United States had lagged behind many other industrial countries

- These policymakers adapted policy for using independent research to inform decisions about drug coverage from countries that offer universal entitlement to health care

- The policymakers countered strong opposition to the new policy from the pharmaceutical industry and its surrogates; even in states that were less rigorous than others in basing coverage decisions on independent research

Because I describe these events as the convergence of science and governance, I begin by defining these three terms. By "science," I mean the international body of independent research evaluating, ever more precisely and persuasively, the effectiveness, comparative effectiveness, and sometimes the cost-effectiveness of interventions to improve health. I accord particular emphasis to the science of research synthesis and to its principal product, systematic reviews, which offer unprecedented rigor in framing research questions, identifying relevant literature and assessing its quality, summarizing evidence, and interpreting findings.

By "governance," I mean what public officials do to, for, and with colleagues in other agencies and branches of government, employees and stakeholders of business and nonprofit organizations, representatives of interest and advocacy groups, and voters. A leading scholar of governance describes it as "a technology of public action with its own history, structures and rationalities."[3]

By "convergence," I mean the use of science in governance: in formal deliberative processes through which state officials and the external advisers they choose collaborate to acquire and use the best available evidence to inform decisions about coverage for health services. For a substantial number of states, convergence also means that policymakers and their advisers are collaborating with researchers selected by public officials to plan, commission, evaluate, and communicate the findings of reviews of evidence of the effectiveness and comparative effectiveness of health services that are conducted according to internationally accepted standards of independence and rigor.

WHY STATES ACTED: IMMEDIATE CAUSES

The convergence described in this book had immediate and underlying causes. The most compelling immediate cause was the recession that began in the spring of 2000 and sharply reduced states' revenues from taxes. This revenue shortfall continued into 2003.

Reducing or even containing the growth of state expenditures for pharmaceutical drugs became a high priority for many policymakers. They mobilized allies in order to deflect challenges from pressure groups, including threats to withhold campaign contributions. Spending for pharmaceutical drugs had been increasing faster than other health costs, which had been growing at double the rate of inflation in the general economy except for a brief pause in the mid-1990s. Because of the recession, policymakers could balance attacks on the new policy for making decisions about covering prescription drugs against demands from other groups advocating, for example, level or increased spending for education, roads, and public transportation.

The damaged reputation of the pharmaceutical industry was another immediate cause of these events. These corporations continued earning large and increasing profits despite the recession. Pharmaceutical manufacturers were charging the highest prices in the world to private employers who offered health coverage to their employees. These prices were often more than federal law permitted them to charge state Medicaid programs. Many manufacturers were also involved in well-publicized scandals about billing fraud, illegal promotion of off-label prescribing, exchanging meals for sales talks, and offering accommodations at lavish resorts ancillary to continuing medical education. Moreover, manufacturers' claims that rising drug prices were mainly a result of the cost of research and development proved to be inaccurate. Data that companies are required to submit to the U.S. Securities and Exchange Commission revealed that most pharmaceutical manufacturers spent more on lobbying and marketing than they did on research. Because of the diminished reputation of the industry, state policymakers could often count on support for, or at least neutrality about, their new coverage policy from leading private employers.

Michigan was the first state to establish the new policy for covering pharmaceutical drugs for enrollees in its Medicaid fee-for-service program. In the spring of 2001, Governor John Engler, a Republican, appointed a committee of physicians and pharmacists to examine evidence from independent research and then recommend for coverage the most effective drugs within each major class. The state would place these drugs on a preferred drug list (PDL) and would pay only the lowest price charged among manufacturers of equally effective drugs. Physicians could prescribe any drug on the list and could request exceptions to prescribe other drugs.

The pharmaceutical industry attacked. Pfizer, a major employer in the state, threatened to close its manufacturing plant in Kalamazoo. Engler then sequestered the committee that was analyzing evidence about the effectiveness of competing drugs in order to protect it from external influence. He also announced that he would not meet with lobbyists for the pharmaceutical industry before the committee reported. The Commissioner of Community Health, James Haveman, held a press conference during which he dumped on a table the contents of a shopping bag that contained one month's gifts and invitations to dine and travel from drug companies to a primary care physician in Grand Rapids. At the request of Engler and Haveman, Tommy Thompson, a former governor of Wisconsin who had recently become secretary of the federal Department of Health and Human

Services, waived Medicaid regulations in order to permit Michigan to establish its PDL. The industry sued Thompson; it eventually lost.[4]

In the fall of 2001, Haveman described these events to colleagues from other states at several meetings of the Reforming States Group (RSG). The RSG, organized in 1991, is a voluntary, nonpartisan association of leaders of the executive and legislative branches of the fifty states and, in recent years, Canadian provinces, Australian states and territories, England, and Scotland. His colleagues asked many questions, especially about the strength of the evidence for choosing preferred drugs and the involvement of leaders of the medical profession in selecting drugs and devising the mechanism by which physicians could request permission to prescribe nonpreferred drugs.

Some members of the RSG had learned about PDLs a year earlier. During its annual Western Regional Meeting in December 2000, John Santa, a member of the staff of Oregon Governor John Kitzhaber, a Democrat, had asked if anyone had information about the science-based Reference Drug Program in the Canadian province of British Columbia. A participant in the meeting (full disclosure: it was me, helping to staff the RSG) said that he had a case study of the program in his laptop, and that Bob Nakagawa, its lead author, was the policymaker who had designed and implemented it.

In February 2001, Nakagawa visited Salem at the invitation of Mark Gibson, Governor Kitzhaber's policy adviser for health and social policy. By midsummer, the Oregon Legislature had enacted a law that permitted the executive branch to create a preferred drug list and required it to assess the effectiveness of competing drugs. The examples of Michigan and British Columbia informed the policy crafted by Gibson and his colleagues.

That fall, Governor Kitzhaber, collaborating with AARP and the Milbank Memorial Fund, an endowed operating foundation based in New York City, convened a two-day open meeting in Portland. In his keynote speech, the governor said that the purpose of the meeting was to discuss ways to "globalize the evidence and localize the policy." Bill Novelli, the chief executive of AARP (formerly the American Association of Retired Persons) endorsed the governor's theme in a second keynote address. Several hundred state officials, lobbyists and experts on health policy from all over the country attended. Andrew D. Oxman, a researcher and public official in Norway, described the methodology of the science of research synthesis and how it was being used to evaluate the quality of studies of primary data and combine the results of acceptable studies in reports called systematic reviews. Oxman and policymakers from Canada and the United Kingdom then described how systematic reviews were informing policy for covering prescription drugs.[5]

Representatives of the pharmaceutical industry criticized systematic reviews and PDLs in the discussion that followed these presentations. They said that systematic reviews were less informative and less rigorous than the well-designed clinical trials conducted by the companies themselves in order to obtain approval to market a drug from the Food and Drug Administration (FDA). Moreover, they said, PDLs would lower the quality of care, because they interfered with patients' and physicians' freedom of choice.

Other participants challenged these arguments. Persons familiar with the research that informed decisions about drug coverage in other countries explained why the findings of systematic reviews had greater statistical power than findings from even the best-designed randomized controlled trials (RCTs). Moreover, most of the trials financed by drug companies compared a new drug with a placebo in order to meet FDA requirements; but evidence about the comparative effectiveness of competing drugs was more useful for making coverage policy. Several participants said that "detailing" to physicians by industry salespersons and direct-to-consumer advertising probably threatened freedom of choice more than science-based coverage policy did.

In 2001 and 2002, in summary, one of the most conservative governors (Engler), and one of the most liberal (Kitzhaber), supported by a former centrist governor now serving in President George W. Bush's cabinet (Thompson), defied the pharmaceutical industry in order to establish policy to use the findings of independent research, and especially systematic reviews, to evaluate competing drugs in order to decide which of them to make available to persons eligible for Medicaid and the State Children's Health Insurance Program. In September 2002, the *Wall Street Journal* reported that "about a dozen" states "use PDLs or are in the process of setting them up," adding: "Michigan officials say its PDL is saving the state $800,000 a week; Louisiana hopes to save $60 million a year."[6]

THE UNDERLYING CAUSES OF CONVERGENCE

Persuasive Research on Fair Tests of Interventions

The rising cost of prescription drugs during a recession and the diminished reputation of the pharmaceutical industry made possible policy to establish PDLs. But this policy had four significant underlying causes. The first was the development and implementation of research methods that, for the first time, permitted fair and persuasive tests of the effectiveness and comparative effectiveness of health services. The second was the representativeness, managerial competence and expertise in health policy of senior officials of state government. The third was frustration among policymakers about their failure to contain the growth of spending for health care. The fourth was the growing burden of chronic disease; a stimulus of increased spending but, equally important, a source of skepticism among policymakers about the priorities of physicians and hospitals and the organization of health services.

To introduce the first of these underlying causes, I return to John Santa's question about policy in British Columbia during the meeting of the RSG in December, 2000. The draft case study was in my computer because Andrew Oxman and I had commissioned case studies of collaboration between policymakers and scientists in six countries in applying the findings of research on the effectiveness of health services. The policymakers and scientists who wrote the case studies had met in Cape Town, South Africa, two months earlier to review one another's drafts and seek consensus about lessons from them for colleagues.[7]

We chose Cape Town for the meeting because half the participants would be there to attend the eighth annual colloquium of the Cochrane Collaboration, the governing body of which Oxman chaired. The Cochrane Collaboration, named in honor of the British epidemiologist Archie Cochrane (1909–88), then comprised about 10,000 persons, mostly researchers, from more than eighty countries. Groups within the Collaboration set standards for systematic reviews, a significant advance in methodology for rigorous evaluation of health services, and then applied them. The Collaboration published the Cochrane Library, an electronic journal of reviews that met its standards, as well as abstracts of reviews in progress. It also supervised a global registry of published and unpublished clinical trials, the sources of primary data for most systematic reviews.[8]

Most of the founders of the Collaboration, like Archie Cochrane himself, had conducted RCTs that were independent of industry. These trials sought to avoid systematic bias in evaluating and comparing interventions through rigorous analysis of data collected from randomly selecting research subjects under procedures that prevented either the subjects or the persons treating them knowing who received which intervention. Trialists, as they called themselves, worried that observational research—mainly the analysis of data from clinical and billing records (called administrative data)—risked several types of bias that could skew findings.

The United States lagged behind most other industrial countries in the priority it accorded, relative to other biomedical and health services research, to conducting independent RCTs and synthesizing their data in systematic reviews. Most of the Americans who studied the outcomes of health interventions used administrative data, of which, as a result of its fragmented payment system, the United States had more than any other country. American researchers devised subtle methods (to adjust for acuity and age, for instance) in order to reduce bias in studying these data. Their studies were generally less expensive and took less time than RCTs.

Americans who conducted independent RCTs had relatively less financial support and considerably lower prestige among health researchers than trialists in, for example, Australia, Canada, Denmark, and the United Kingdom. The National Institutes of Health and its most powerful constituents in academic medicine resisted the deflection or reallocation of funds from research on the pathophysiology of disease to independent RCTs. They did so mainly because they believed that research in the basic health sciences and traditional clinical investigation would lead more rapidly to improvements in population health than evaluation of the effectiveness of interventions. Moreover, the federal agencies and the few philanthropic foundations that sponsored research on health services had many competing demands on their budgets.

Many academic researchers, including those who evaluated health services, had other reasons to be critical of RCTs. They were expensive, time-consuming and often difficult to conduct. RCTs could violate ethical principles; especially if potentially effective treatment was withheld for the sake of comparison. Moreover, most RCTs evaluated interventions in carefully chosen patients in academic settings rather than in routine practice.

Many researchers also disparaged RCTs because they associated them with commercial interests. Pharmaceutical companies sponsored most American RCTs in order to obtain regulatory approval for new drugs. Many senior investigators at academic health centers had low regard for colleagues who administered research protocols that had been designed by pharmaceutical companies and then published articles about the trials that had been ghostwritten by company staff or contractors. Since the early 1990s, moreover, private firms had been conducting an increasing number of industry-sponsored trials, thus reducing still further their prestige among academic scientists.

A growing number of leaders in the legislative and executive branches of government in American states had, however, been learning about the methods, strengths, uses and limitations of independent RCTs and systematic reviews since 1990. By 2000, when approximately 2,500 systematic reviews that met the methodological standards of the Cochrane Collaboration had been published, a substantial number of influential policymakers understood how RCTs and systematic reviews could contribute to policy for coverage and for quality improvement; if, that is, it became politically feasible to use them.

These policymakers initially learned about the methods, strengths, uses and limitations of what came to be called, oversimply, evidence-based health research as a result of the work of the User Liaison Program (ULP) of the federal Agency for Health Care Research and Policy (now the Agency for Healthcare Research and Quality or AHRQ) and the Milbank Memorial Fund. Between its inception in 1976 and 1991, ULP had organized interactive workshops at which state (and some local) government policymakers learned about the methods and uses of research on health services. Until 1990 most of the research described in ULP workshops was observational; the methods and findings of investigators who used administrative data to study variation in the services offered to patients and the outcomes of treatment. I had helped to organize and defend ULP as a federal official and was subsequently a planner, presenter, and facilitator for many of its workshops. The Milbank Memorial Fund appointed me its president in the fall of 1989.

Because of the work of ULP and Milbank, state policymakers learned about the methods and uses of RCTs and systematic reviews conducted in other countries. At the end of 1989, Iain Chalmers, a Scot based in Oxford, published, with collaborators principally from Canada and the Netherlands, two volumes on *Effective Care in Pregnancy and Childbirth*.[9] This was the first demonstration that systematic reviews could be used to evaluate an entire field of health care. Three years later Chalmers, who had been close to Archie Cochrane, was the principal organizer of the Collaboration.

Chalmers showed me the volumes in January 1990. I paged through them as he talked about his plans to organize an international collaborative network of investigators who would conduct systematic reviews of health services. At the end of the second volume, I found several appendices; lists of interventions of proven effectiveness; of those that should be discontinued; and of others with uncertain effects that required further research.

Several months later, the director of ULP asked me to help plan and then lead the closing session of a three-day workshop for some forty state policymakers about research on the outcomes of health services. When my turn came, I asked the participants to assume for a moment that the slides I would now show them listed findings that met the highest international standards for research. I promised that I would describe the methodology of this research after they had responded to the slides.

My slides were the first pages of each of the appendices of *Effective Care in Pregnancy and Childbirth*. But when I spoke I changed the scientific language that Chalmers and his colleagues had used to describe each list. I said that the slides could be headed stop doing this, do that differently, cover these interventions when you have extra money, and do more research.

Most of the policymakers in the room said they were intrigued. Lee Greenfield, then chair of the committee of the Minnesota House of Representatives that financed health services and public health, called the lists "an answer to a policymaker's prayer;" depending, he added, on the persuasiveness of the methodology on which they were based. Greenfield had studied physics and engineering at Purdue and the philosophy of science at the University of Minnesota.

A conference in Washington, DC, early in 1991 contributed additional evidence that systematic reviews and research that met rigorous criteria for inclusion in them could help to improve the effectiveness of health services. The International Association for Healthcare Technology Assessment (now Health Technology Assessment International), several federal agencies, the American College of Obstetrics and Gynecology and the Milbank Memorial Fund convened the conference to discuss the significance of *Effective Care in Pregnancy and Childbirth*. Several hundred participants heard presentations about systematic reviews and how they could be used to improve clinical and financing policy for perinatal care. In a keynote speech, the senior health official in the federal government, Assistant Secretary of Health James Mason, endorsed the science of research synthesis and its applications.

Early in 1993 a cover story in *Parade* described the benefits to consumers of the findings and methods of *Effective Care in Pregnancy and Childbirth*. Earl Ubell, a senior editor at the magazine who had been a pioneering science reporter on network television, instigated and wrote the story.[10] Ubell quoted me in the second jump, which was buried among classified advertisements. By the next morning, however, the voice mailbox at the Milbank Fund had received many inquiries from women all over the country wanting to know more about the book.

Because the Fund's mission is to help decisionmakers apply the best available evidence and experience in order to improve health policy, its response to these consumers was to tell them how to acquire the paperback condensation of the book. Fund staff then began a multi-year initiative to inform policymakers about the methods and potential uses of systematic reviews.

The Competence of State Government

The second underlying cause of convergence was the competence of senior state officials in making health policy. Legislative leaders and members of their staff, governors and persons they appointed led in developing this competence over many years. I call these people "general government" in order to distinguish their responsibilities from those of persons I call "specialized government." General government allocates resources among competing claimants, who include agencies of the executive branches, public benefit corporations, local government, interest groups, and citizens. Specialized government advocates; its employees compete to increase the resources allocated to their agencies by general government, at whose expense is not their concern. General government made convergence possible.

Many historians, journalists, and political scientists, as well as many federal officials, have argued since the late nineteenth century that states hindered the inevitable centralization of the economy and domestic policy. Many of these critics also complained about the incompetence and dishonesty of state officials. But state officials were never as irrelevant or as incompetent as their detractors claimed. Moreover, government in the states has become increasingly effective since World War II in response to growing responsibilities and spending to fulfill them, especially in health affairs.

The vast expansion of public higher education for the health professions after 1945 drew state officials into other aspects of health policy. States had for more than a century been responsible for public health, for inpatient treatment for persons who were mentally ill and disabled, for inspecting hospitals and, in many states, for supplementing charity in paying for the care of the indigent. By the late 1940s, states were subsidizing capital and appropriating operating funds to build and expand public and nonprofit teaching hospitals. State officials were leading participants in implementing an internationally accepted theory that population health would improve if health care were organized in hierarchical pyramids topped by academic institutions and clinical facilities they controlled.[11]

This theory, which I call hierarchical regionalism, also influenced legislation in 1946 establishing the federal Hill-Burton program to construct hospitals. Because Hill-Burton funds flowed in response to state plans, states' responsibilities for inpatient care expanded beyond the hospitals they owned or whose capital they subsidized.

Because of Hill-Burton and other federal grant programs, every state expanded the size and sophistication of its civil service in order to comply with federal regulations for reporting and accounting. The extramural program of the National Institutes of Health, for example, began to award grants in 1946; many of them to state universities. Within a few years, states also received new federal funds to provide financial support to poor children and elderly persons and for payments to vendors of health services to these populations.

States' responsibilities in health affairs grew as the health sector expanded. They regulated many more hospitals and nursing homes, whether public, nonprofit, or proprietary. They oversaw the construction and expansion of health facilities and provided increasing amounts of subsidized capital to nonprofit hospitals and nursing homes. As enrolment in voluntary health insurance plans increased, so did states' responsibility to regulate the solvency, market conduct, and products of the commercial and nonprofit firms that sold it. The insurance industry persuaded Congress to pass a law that clarified and strengthened states' authority to regulate insurance, even companies in interstate commerce.

Many experts in universities, research organizations, and the federal government continued to proclaim the inevitability of greater centralization in the decades after World War II. For many academic political scientists, centralization was the domestic counterpart to the increased power of the presidency in foreign and defense policy. They adduced evidence from the poorest (which were also, not coincidentally, the most defiantly racist) states to support their claim that states would (and should) wither away. Generations of students of American government learned that the "Alabama problem" was an example of the need to centralize domestic policy.

Only a few proponents of the inevitability of centralization noticed the consequences for state government of changes in where people lived. Mainly as a result of employment opportunities during and after World War II, many people, both black and white, migrated from the South and border states to the Northeast, Midwest, and Pacific West. Many African Americans had their first opportunity to participate in politics; many whites had a choice among competing candidates for public office for the first time.

Many people from the Midwest, Mid-Atlantic, and New England states also moved, seeking jobs and a more benign climate, to metropolitan regions in the South and Southwest. Many of these migrants had higher expectations about the scope and efficiency of public services than many of their new neighbors.

The prosperity of mobile Americans stimulated the growth of suburbs and of the influence of their residents on state politics and government.[12] Most of the new suburbanites were homeowners who held mid-level jobs in the public and private sectors. They wanted a great deal from government, including schools and universities that would increase their children's opportunities, roads, bridges, and in some places mass transit that would reduce the time they spent commuting and shopping, hospitals that had the latest technology and offered rapid access in emergencies, and zoning that enhanced or at least protected the value of their homes. Many of them were willing to pay more state and local taxes to achieve these benefits. They began to elect people like themselves to legislatures.

The U.S. Supreme Court soon helped to redistribute political power in the states from rural areas to suburbs. Most state legislatures had traditionally established the boundaries of districts for electing their members and members of the U.S. Congress in ways that skewed power to voters in rural areas. This situation changed rapidly after 1962 when, in two landmark decisions, the U.S. Supreme Court established and then applied the constitutional principle of one person, one vote.

The characteristics of legislators changed after states redistricted. Many of the new legislators from urban and suburban districts had more education, and more of them were professionals, women, and members of minority racial, religious, and ethnic groups than many of their rural predecessors.

Redistricting coincided with the expansion of public spending for health by the federal government and the states as a result of the enactment of Medicare and Medicaid in 1965. Medicaid was a federal-state program. Medicare, although entirely a federal program, combined with Medicaid to transform the financing of hospital and medical services for the poor and for elderly persons with modest incomes. Patients whose care had previously been subsidized by government and philanthropy became significant, and often the most prompt and reliable, sources of reimbursement for hospitals and physicians.

State officials were now responsible for access to appropriate care for a huge percentage of the population. They continued to regulate hospitals, nursing homes, and health insurance, to subsidize care in teaching hospitals, and to provide care for special populations. Now states also had responsibility for patients covered by Medicaid for acute and long-term care, and shared with the federal government responsibility for seniors and persons with disabilities whose low incomes entitled them to both Medicaid and Medicare.

States' spending for health, including public health activities and education and training for the health professions, became a huge percentage of their budgets. Medicaid became a larger budget item than education in many states. States that deinstitutionalized most services for persons who were mentally ill and developmentally disabled could, under federal regulations, substitute Medicaid for what had been state-only funding. Moreover, Medicaid became the largest payer for long-term care. Because of "spend down" provisions to implement the legal construct of "medical indigence," long-term care became an entitlement for people with higher income and more assets than other Medicaid recipients.

Increased Spending, Uncertain Revenue

Spending for health services, in total dollars and as a percentage of gross national product, has grown in every industrial country during the past half century, but most rapidly in the United States. Expenditures for health services for the first time exceeded spending for national defense during the 1960s. In most subsequent years, the rate of inflation in spending for health services has exceeded the rate of general inflation.

High expenditures for health services in the United States have many causes. The most important drivers of spending have been the introduction of new technology and the weakness of policy to restrain its proliferation. A related source of spending growth has been the overuse and misuse of some of this technology and the underuse of less expensive preventive and primary care services. Some of the increase is, moreover, a result of disease mongering by manufacturers of drugs and their allies among providers; the medicalization, for example, of anxiety, sadness, and stress. Much of the inflation has also resulted from the administrative complexity of billing and reimbursing for services in a sector with many public and private payers. Very little of the increase, however, is the result of the aging of the population; a counterintuitive finding first recognized in European countries and recently confirmed in the United States by the Congressional Budget Office.[13]

Much of the increased spending has been beneficial. More people have had access to more health services in recent decades than at any time in the past. Although there is strong evidence that increasing length of life over the past century has mainly been a result of other determinants of health than personal health services, advances in diagnostic, preventive, and therapeutic technologies have had a significant effect on both the length and quality of life.[14]

As health care became the largest sector of the American economy, increasing payments by government, health insurance plans and consumers generated considerable personal and corporate income. Pressure from interest groups whose members benefited from rising expenditures has made it easier for policymakers in the states and the federal government to increase the supply of services than to restrain spending for redundant and ineffective services in order to subsidize access to essential care for more people.

Rising expenditure for health services has placed an increasing burden on the states, the federal government, and business firms. Expenditure growth is a particular problem for states because their annual revenue from taxes and fees varies within each business cycle, while their constitutions, with the exception of Vermont's, require them to balance their budgets annually.

Policymakers in the public and private sectors have tried to restrain spending in a variety of ways. Their strategies have included capping and freezing reimbursement to institutions and professionals; encouraging competition among providers; requiring prior approval for patients to receive drugs and surgery; limiting patients' coverage and raising deductibles and copayments; reducing or refusing to increase educational opportunities for aspirants to the health professions; and restraining the building and expansion of facilities.

Interest groups threatened by each of these strategies have complained that they compromise patients' access to health care of the highest quality. Policy for spending less, increasing spending more slowly, and spending better became inseparable from policy for access and quality. Any proposal for policy to restrain spending stimulated debate about access and quality. Similarly, any policy to address quality stimulated charges by interest groups and advocates that it was a covert attempt to reduce spending.

Physicians and the organizations that represent them have since the 1920s interpreted most proposed policy to address access, quality, and cost (defined as spending that they ordered for particular patients) as threats to their professional autonomy. Because many of these proposals have been informed by research on health services, most physicians and the organizations that represent them have been severe critics of the methods and findings of such research. This criticism has affected funding for the field, researchers' careers, and the framing of questions for research.

The politics of physicians' autonomy has profoundly affected the history of convergence. The legislation that established Medicare and Medicaid in 1965 accorded considerable autonomy to physicians in both treating patients and setting fees. The politics of cost containment over the next half century diminished but never eliminated this autonomy. The preferred drug lists (PDLs) that are the focus of this book, for example, substitute policy informed by independent research for physician autonomy in prescribing drugs. PDLs are an aspect of a gradual process by which public officials and corporate executives have become less solicitous of physicians' preferences.

Although physicians and many of the associations that represent them still use the rhetoric of autonomy, the politics of medicine is changing. Leaders of the major associations of the profession (who call themselves the House of Medicine) have explored strategies to preserve substantial autonomy by accepting more accountability to government and private employers. These leaders are promising increased accountability to the public for the quality and safety of medical practice in exchange for the profession's continued dominance of medical education, licensure and discipline, and specialty certification. Nevertheless, the politics of medical autonomy still has substantial influence on policymaking to restrain spending and improve quality.

Chronic Disease and the Inefficiency of Health Care Delivery

Until roughly the 1960s, it seemed reasonable to most people that public and private sector coverage should accord the highest priority to resource-intensive care during acute episodes of illness, whether patients suffered such episodes as a result of infections, injuries, or chronic disease. Since the early twentieth century, there had been consensus that the principal determinants of life and death were whether, how promptly, and how effectively providers of health services addressed these episodes. Because hospitals provided the most effective care during acute episodes it was logical for policymakers to prioritize increasing the supply of hospital and specialized services rather than of primary care. Similarly, payers reimbursed providers more generously for inpatient than for ambulatory care, and particularly for invasive procedures. Few diseases could be prevented by medical intervention until after mid-century. Moreover, only a few drugs cured infections or slowed the course of chronic disease before the 1940s.[15]

A widely accepted assumption about biomedical science reinforced for many years the priority accorded to treating acute episodes of illness. Most scientists, journalists, and members of the public assumed that the germ theory of infectious disease would be the model for understanding the natural history of chronic disease, and thus of research to prevent and eventually to cure it. The microscopic agents that caused chronic disease would be isolated in laboratories. Physicians who worked in laboratories and treated patients, assisted by scientists in other disciplines, would devise simple preventive measures and cures. These interventions were sometimes called, usually admiringly, "magic bullets" during and even after the first half of the twentieth century. Magic bullets would proliferate and gradually lead to improvement in the health of populations. As recently as 1971, for example, an influential medical scientist and pundit disparaged interventions that merely postponed death rather than curing disease as "half-way technologies."[16]

Chronic disease became the leading cause of death in the United States by the 1920s. In the mid-1930s, a cross section of Americans told federal surveyors that their most important health concern was mitigating the disabling effects of chronic disease. But health policy continued to prioritize interventions during acute episodes of disease. The few effective interventions for chronic disease seemed to be magic bullets, notably, insulin treatment for diabetes and vitamin therapy for pernicious anemia. Surgeons were intervening more effectively, especially to treat cancers. Chronic disease, most experts had reason to believe, would eventually yield to drugs and surgery.

A few epidemiologists and medical scientists had, however, begun in the 1920s to array evidence that chronic disease presented different challenges for research, practice, and policy than infectious disease. Working in laboratories and applying advances in statistical methods, they demonstrated that chronic diseases had a variety of causes, often linked, which included bacteria, viruses, genes, environmental toxins, personal behavior, injuries, and the biology of aging. This research eventually established the conceptual basis for policy and practice to prevent or delay acute episodes of chronic disease and alleviate pain and other symptoms through more effective management of patients' disease. Prevention, research indicated, should also include reducing environmental hazards, particularly those resulting from industrial processes, and persuading people to modify their behavior.

Policy for health services accommodated gradually to the growing prevalence of chronic disease. Hierarchical regionalism, the dominant theory of the organization of services, had been devised early in the twentieth century to treat infectious disease and casualties of war. The politics of physicians' autonomy thwarted hierarchical regionalism in the United States. These politics also gave community hospitals and the specialists who practiced in them financial incentives to treat acute episodes of chronic disease. Most of these physicians, as well as public and private payers, were slow to implement advances in managing care for chronic disease in outpatient settings.

During the first decade after World War II, the priorities of health policy and Americans' experience of illness diverged more widely than at any time before or since. Americans had more chronic disease and hence suffered more disability than ever before. As a result of the growth of employment-based health insurance, they also had more access than ever before to more care for infectious disease, injuries, and acute episodes of chronic disease. New government subsidies increased the supply of acute care hospital services and offered advanced training to more specialists, especially in invasive disciplines, than to primary care physicians.

Beginning in the mid-1950s, health policy began to accommodate to the prevalence of chronic disease and advances in preventing and managing it. Major medical insurance, devised by commercial insurers, paid for and coordinated expensive outpatient and hospital care for chronic disease in exchange for higher deductibles and co-insurance. A decade later, Medicare began to reimburse more services for managing chronic disease than any previous insurance program, public or private. In 1972, the federal government extended Medicare coverage to persons eligible for Social Security Disability Insurance (which had been established in 1956) and socialized the cost of treating end-stage renal disease. Medicaid subsidized a vast increase in the availability of skilled nursing facilities and home health care.

A few reformers insisted that despite these incremental changes in the allocation of resources, the organization of health services and reimbursement for them required radical reform. They argued that, in the absence of major changes in how and where physicians practiced and how they applied evidence about the effectiveness of interventions, health spending would rise more quickly than necessary. Moreover, the outcomes of care would not justify these expenditures.

Leaders of many powerful interest groups in health affairs agreed that the delivery system and reimbursement policy should accommodate to the prevalence of chronic disease. But they also represented their members and constituents. Specialists in surgery, interventional subspecialties of internal medicine, and radiology continued to be more highly paid than their colleagues who managed the chronic disease of their patients. Episodic management of patients' diseases and overprescribing of tests, drugs, and invasive treatment continued.

Many officials of general government in the states acknowledged serious flaws in the organization of health services. They knew that many hospitals were overequipped and underutilized and that government agencies and private health insurance plans reimbursed physicians for many procedures of dubious effectiveness. Voters frequently complained to them about their lack of access to primary care. Officials observed that much of the increased spending on prescription drugs was a result of overprescribing, often in response to demand generated among physicians and consumers by pharmaceutical companies. Many of them talked to one another about the excess suffering and waste of resources that resulted from services that were inefficient and ineffective. The convergence of science and governance described in this book became a small, but significant, way to address some of these problems.

HOW THIS BOOK IS ORGANIZED

The chapters that follow amplify and continue through the spring of 2009 the stories I have summarized in the preceding pages. The next chapter describes how the politics of health policy has shaped the scope, priorities, and methods of research on health services. This chapter begins in the early twentieth century in order to document the persisting influence of past politics on subsequent events; particularly the politics of asserting, defending and negotiating the autonomy of the medical profession.

The subject of Chapter 3 is how and why leaders of state government became receptive to research on health services and especially to the research that makes convergence possible. The chapter describes the growing capacity of states in making and implementing policy; initially for public health, then for higher education for the health professions, and since the 1950s, for personal health services.

Chapter 4 describes the convergence of science and governance in American states through a history of the origin, work, and effects of the Drug Effectiveness Review Project (DERP). The chapter describes the process of mutual assistance that DERP's member states and a Canadian intergovernmental organization devised and how researchers and state officials collaborate to produce systematic reviews. The history of health services research and of state government in health policy described in the preceding chapters made DERP possible. Immediate events and underlying causes made it feasible. Particular policymakers and their staff made DERP happen.

The final chapter assesses the sustainability of the convergence of science and governance exemplified by DERP. It emphasizes the fragility that threatens the partial success to date. The chapter also raises issues that policymakers and researchers could address as they prepare for contingencies that either threaten convergence or offer opportunities to expand it.

A COMMENT ON SOURCES AND METHODS

Many of the sources for this book could be described in conventional scholarly language: interviews, participant observation, published primary and secondary sources (articles in print and electronic media, publications by researchers), published documents (reports, bills, laws, court decisions) and unpublished documents (letters, e-mail messages, internal memoranda, draft legislation and regulations, legal briefs).

These conventional words misstate how I acquired most of my sources. My "interviews" were mainly privileged conversations with policymakers and researchers. I was a "participant observer" because I had to listen attentively (and consider my responses carefully) in order to offer advice that policymakers might find useful or to assist them in drafting memoranda, legislative specifications, budget documents, and official publications. I had access to unpublished documents about politics and policy—documents that would subsequently be deposited in archives—because they were part of my daily work with colleagues in government. I read published sources because policymakers asked me to or because reading them was preparation for what policymakers might ask me to do.

I have been talking with policymakers and members of their staff and reading internal and published documents on the subjects I address in this book for four decades. I have been fortunate to experience public life in quite different environments and thus to learn about the priorities, processes, and predilections of people who work in them. These environments include three federal agencies, government in two states, two universities, and an endowed operating foundation.

As a result of how I acquired information, I have different ethical obligations than most scholars who write about politics and policy. I did not seek informed consent before engaging in any of the conversations that inform this book. I had access to confidential information because policymakers and their staff as well as colleagues in the field of health services research assumed that I could be trusted. Many of the primary data in this book were confidential until released by the persons who provided them.

For many years I have solicited comments on excerpts from and sometimes entire drafts of articles and book chapters from the policymakers whose experience I report and interpret. I invite them to request complete anonymity or imprecise attribution for any quotation or paraphrase of what they say. I also promise to take account of each comment they make about how I interpret their statements or behavior.

I stipulate, however, that taking account of comments does not necessarily mean that I will change my interpretation of sources. A co-author and I once revised the conclusion of an article to add that a former policymaker took exception to our interpretation of his purpose in crafting an amendment to the Internal Revenue Code. We revised again when the policymaker wrote us that, on reflection, he agreed with our interpretation.[17]

The citations in this book reflect this interpretation of my ethical obligations. I cite published and archival sources in the conventional way. Whether I name an informant or attribute a quotation or an anecdote by title (for example, to a committee chair, a senator, or the executive of a professional association), I usually do not provide the precise date or setting of the comment. I omit this information in order to enable my colleagues in public service to maintain ownership of information about what they said to whom, where, when, and under what circumstances. The absence of a citation signifies that my source chose anonymity.

I am sometimes the source of an uncited quotation, paraphrase, or description of an event. I identify myself as a source only when I am a character in a story. In this chapter, for example, I described why I had a draft case study of the PDL in British Columbia when a state official asked about that policy and my role in introducing systematic reviews to state policymakers. When my presence did not affect a story, however, I report, without attribution, what I heard. In borderline cases, when my presence had only a modest affect, I usually choose anonymity in order to maintain narrative focus on more important characters.

I hope my strategy for describing and citing sources also meets my ethical obligations to persons whose permission to quote or paraphrase them I did not seek. These people made ill-considered, or deliberately misleading, or self-serving, or merely outrageous comments in conversation with me or at a meeting I attended. I have tried to prevent even the most knowledgeable readers from identifying these sources.

Another ethical issue is my decision not to discuss with policymakers my interpretations of the causes of political events. To do so would impose the preoccupations of scholars on people who have other interests and many demands on their time. Only once during my career has a policymaker found and read a book I wrote and commended it to colleagues.

I have sometimes, however, told a few policymakers about interpretations of mine that academic colleagues have dismissed. Each time the policymakers replied that my interpretation was obvious to them. An example is the distinction between general and special government introduced in this chapter and elaborated in Chapter 3.

In contrast to my reticence about discussing interpretation with policymakers, I have asked many of them about the political and financial costs and potential benefits of many policies. That is their business, and I am grateful for their guidance, which is, I hope, reflected in this book.

My greatest ethical regret is that the conventions of writing a book require me to imply that the politics of policymaking is more coherent than it actually is. Much of what I ascribe to causation could also be interpreted as responses to contingency.

2. Research on Health Services and the Politics of Health

Findings from research on health services have only recently begun routinely to inform aspects of health policy in the United States. But the systematic study of health services has informed and been informed by health politics and policy for a century. This chapter and the next, on state government and health policy, seek to explain why some researchers and some state officials were prepared by the end of the 1990s to do the work that I call convergence.

Since the early twentieth century, considerable research has examined who, trained and organized how, delivers what health services to whom, at what cost, paid by whom, and with what effects. Researchers who studied these issues have included persons who began their careers working primarily as clinicians and clinical teachers, basic scientists, statisticians, epidemiologists, public health officials, operations researchers, economists, sociologists, political scientists, and anthropologists. Many of them continued to identify with these disciplines. The boundaries separating clinical, public health, and what in the 1960s began to be called health services research, have always been blurred. This chapter focuses on research, usually conducted at or near these boundaries, which addressed controversial political issues.

The most powerful people in health affairs, supported by the media and much of the public, have accorded lower priority to the study of health services than to other areas of health research. For more than a century, prevailing opinion, translated into policy, has ascribed most advances in the health of the public to research in the basic biological sciences and its application to the study of the natural history of disease, its transmission, acquisition, burden, and the mechanisms by which vaccines, drugs and procedures affect its course. An alternative opinion, that there are broader determinants of health and longevity, has had much less influence on the allocation of resources to and within the health sector. Neither opinion accorded high priority to research on the accessibility, organization, efficiency and effectiveness of health services.

RESEARCH AND HEALTH POLITICS, 1910–1945

Despite its low status relative to other forms of inquiry in the health sector, research on health services has a long history of addressing controversial issues. In 1910, for example, the Carnegie Foundation for the Advancement of Teaching, collaborating with reformers in the American Medical Association (AMA), commissioned Abraham Flexner to evaluate medical schools in the United States and Canada. Flexner based his criteria for evaluation on the policies of the medical school and hospital at the Johns Hopkins University. The faculty at Hopkins had begun in the 1890s to implement innovations in organizing and teaching basic science and clinical disciplines that had been devised in Europe. Flexner found most of the schools he visited deficient on these criteria, which displeased many academic and community physicians and attracted considerable media attention. His report contributed to the closing of a substantial number of schools and the reorganization of most of those that remained.[1]

Controversy also arose about research sponsored by foundations and government to support programs to prevent and treat particular diseases. Beginning in 1912, the Rockefeller Sanitary Commission for the Eradication of Hookworm evaluated the effectiveness of local public health agencies in the South in eliminating the direct causes of the disease. Advocates of higher wages in cotton mills deplored lack of attention to inadequate income and housing as underlying causes of hookworm. In contrast, research by staff of the U.S. Public Health Service (PHS) on reducing the incidence of pellagra pleased reformers, because it identified broader interventions than clinical services. The PHS's Joseph Goldberger and Edgar Sydenstricker concluded in 1915 that the primary cause of pellagra was "uncertain conditions of an economic character."[2]

Controversy about research on health services grew along with the application of its findings. Many physicians and their associations, for example, resisted efforts by the Carnegie and Rockefeller philanthropies to implement the findings of Flexner's research by creating regional hierarchies of health services. Other Rockefeller staff distressed the AMA and state medical societies by documenting that physicians were unevenly distributed in relation to population. Michael Davis, working for various

philanthropic organizations, displeased some public officials by documenting immigrants' lack of access to health care. He also antagonized some
physicians by applying the methods of the emerging field of management
science to the organization of outpatient clinics.[3]

The political implications of research on health services became news-
worthy in the late 1920s and early 1930s as a result of disputed reports
and recommendations of the Committee on the Costs of Medical Care
(CCMC). Seven philanthropic foundations, initially with the cooperation
of the AMA, created the CCMC in 1927 in order to address what a later
generation would call problems of access and quality in the health sector.
A year later, President Herbert Hoover appointed its chairman as secretary
of the interior, the department that then supervised the PHS.[4]

CCMC staff conducted extensive research on health services. For
example, they prepared the first estimate of total health expenditures in
the United States and documented disparities in the distribution of medical
care by geography and income. They also devised standards of good
medical practice based on a national survey of leading medical specialists.
Then they applied these standards to recommend a ratio of acute hospital
beds to population that influenced policy in the federal government and
the states for the next four decades.

A majority of CCMC members and many of its research staff were also
advocates for substantial policy reform. In its final report late in 1932, the
Committee adopted recommendations that appalled most physicians. A
minority of the Committee, including the physicians appointed by the
AMA, dissented.

Three recommendations threatened physicians' professional autonomy.
First, that they should be organized in multi-specialty groups that coordinated with hospitals. Second, that medical and hospital services should
be arrayed in hierarchies based on technical complexity within geographi-
cal regions, with academic centers at the apex of each hierarchy. Third,
that payment for health services should be administered by insurance
companies and public agencies, which they called "third parties." The
majority of the CCMC claimed that research findings supported
these recommendations.[5]

Leaders of the AMA and state medical societies and editors of the
medical press protested that the CCMC's recommendations, like the academic imperialism the foundations promoted, were bad policy based on
bad research. Moreover, the CCMC majority represented the same coalition of academics, public health specialists and social science researchers
that had antagonized the profession during attempts a decade earlier to

legislate compulsory health insurance in many states. The recommendations, medical spokespersons said, would prevent individual physicians from choosing appropriate treatment for each of their patients, from being accountable to their peers for the quality of their practice, and from charging fees based on what their colleagues charged and patients could bear.

The Milbank Memorial Fund, a co-sponsor of the CCMC, provided opponents of the recommendations with additional evidence that research on health services threatened their interests. Edgar Sydenstricker, a member of the CCMC, had left the PHS to become the Fund's research director. He dissented from the majority report because it was insufficiently reformist. The Fund's chief executive, John Kingsbury, made speeches and wrote articles supporting reform and claiming that research justified it. Early in 1933, moreover, the Fund hired a former member (Michael Davis) and the deputy research director of CCMC (I. S. Falk). A few months later, Harry Hopkins, President Franklin Roosevelt's principal adviser on unemployment relief and social policy, asked Kingsbury to lend Davis and Falk to serve as health staff to the cabinet committee that was drafting what became the Social Security Act of 1935. Roosevelt was disinclined to challenge organized medicine on health insurance because he feared it would also attack old-age pensions. Hopkins told Kingsbury that he wanted his help in changing the president's mind.[6]

Organized medicine targeted the Fund. Because stock in the Borden Company was the largest holding in the Fund's portfolio, state medical societies asked their members to advise nursing mothers not to use its condensed milk in infant formula.

The Fund also offended organized medicine and its allies in the business community by commissioning Sir Arthur Newsholme, a retired senior health official in Britain, to describe and evaluate the organization and financing of health services in European countries. Newsholme and Kingsbury further enraged critics of health reform by visiting the Soviet Union and then publishing a book, *Red Medicine: Socialized Health in Soviet Russia* (1933), in which they praised health services in that country. The book was illustrated with photographs of happy patients and health staff by Margaret Bourke White, a well-known photojournalist.

Falk and Davis continued to demonstrate that they were avid reformers as well as researchers. As research director for the new Social Security Board (later the Social Security Administration), Falk became a target for antagonists of public funding to increase access to health services and of the welfare state more generally. In 1938, moreover, he helped dissuade the Roosevelt Administration from accepting an offer from the AMA to exchange support for subsidizing hospital construction and improved access to health services for some persons with low incomes for the Administration's silence about health insurance reform.[7] Michael Davis continued to use evidence from research to justify reform in many publications and as an executive of the Rosenwald Fund, a self-liquidating foundation established by the founder of Sears Roebuck.

Organized medicine also tried to suppress publication of research on health services that contradicted its interests. In 1937, for example, Milton Friedman, later in his career a Nobel laureate in Economic Science, completed a doctoral dissertation in which he found that physicians charged higher fees than practitioners of other professions because they controlled entry into medicine. The National Bureau of Economic Research, which employed Friedman when he did this research, mollified the AMA by delaying its publication until 1945. Friedman subsequently proposed the abolition of state licensure of physicians in order to end their monopoly of medical services.[8]

The AMA also commissioned research on health services in order to disparage proposals for reform. Soon after publication of the CCMC report, it created a Bureau of Medical Economics, which was led by Frank G. Dickinson, a former professor at Northwestern University. The AMA's economists found, for example, that because the supply of physicians satisfied demand for their services, it was unnecessary to increase enrolment in medical schools.[9]

The association between research on health services and health policy reform inhibited growth of the field. Most health foundations did not sponsor it again before the 1970s. Until the 1960s, very few academics in the social sciences, clinical medical disciplines, or public health, studied health services; many of the few who did also advocated reform of the organization and financing of care.

Staff of the PHS who studied health services in the 1930s and 1940s also identified with reform. For example, they conducted the landmark National Health Inventory of 1934–35, a survey of a random sample of almost three million people.[10] The survey documented the growing prevalence of chronic disease. In an article based on the survey, its principal investigator began cautiously, emphasizing "population trends and problems of public health." But he concluded by recommending public policy to expand access to care.[11] Other PHS researchers used methodology that had been devised by the CCMC to predict a postwar shortage of physicians, which displeased the AMA, as well as a need for more hospital beds, which the Association applauded. PHS researchers collaborated with staff of the

American Hospital Association to devise a plan for regionalizing hospitals and incorporated it in official documents justifying legislation enacted as the Hill-Burton Hospital Construction Act of 1946.[12] The PHS assigned Milton Roemer to "plan for the implementation of national health insurance should the Wagner-Murray-Dingell Bill be enacted." Roemer soon took a government job in the Canadian province of Saskatchewan after the State Department confiscated his passport because of his membership in left-wing organizations.[13]

Only a few researchers in the first third of the century evaluated the effectiveness of interventions to prevent, diagnose, and treat disease. Most persons who studied health services shared the general opinion that advances in biomedical research conducted in laboratories were the major source of interventions to prevent and treat disease. Relatively few of them challenged the consensus that research in the basic health sciences deserved more funding than clinical research that combined laboratory investigation with the observation of patients. The foundations and pharmaceutical companies that sponsored most medical research before World War II, as well as the NIH, prioritized the study of cell biology, biochemistry, molecular microbiology, physiology, experimental pathology, and pharmacology.

Investigators who combined observation of patients with laboratory research had begun to create a distinct scientific field in the second decade of the century. In the 1920s, for example, Alfred Cohn of the Rockefeller Institute for Medical Research used the methods of the new clinical research to establish chronic heart disease as a condition different from rheumatic fever.[14]

Cohn and most other clinical investigators assumed that applying findings from laboratory work in studies of the course of disease and the effects of treatments in a small number of patients could be translated directly into practice and teaching in regionalized hierarchies of hospitals and medical practices. In order to demonstrate such translation on a large scale, researchers from a consortium of medical schools and their teaching hospitals in New York City established a center for clinical research on chronic disease at a public hospital on Welfare [now Roosevelt] Island in the late 1930s. The Rockefeller Foundation, the Metropolitan Life Insurance Company, and New York City government financed the center.[15]

These funders shared the researchers' assumption that work in laboratories and clinics would lead physicians, as rational devotees of science, to offer more effective services. The Rockefeller Foundation wanted to stimulate applications of findings from its program of research in the basic sciences. The city's commissioner of hospitals expected the presence of the center and its researchers to improve the quality of services and the training of house staff. The statisticians and social scientists at Metropolitan Life, who were among the best-known researchers on health services of their generation, endorsed the center because they expected research on chronic disease to lead to new health insurance products that offered broader coverage than hospitalization for acute episodes of illness. Although Metropolitan Life had financed community nursing services and conducted research that found they prevented premature deaths (and hence postponed life insurance claims) and had sponsored "perhaps the first cooperative controlled trial [in a large population] in this country," company staff were convinced that basic science and clinical research on small populations were the best sources of effective care.[16]

Most advocates of radical reform in the organization and financing of health services agreed that the findings of basic and clinical research would improve health. A historian recently concluded that the reformers "shared a heroic view of scientific progress and medical treatment."[17] They differed from their political adversaries because they reasoned that such reforms as multi-specialty group practice, pre-payment by third parties, and universal coverage would speed the dissemination of beneficial technologies to practicing physicians and hence to a growing number of patients.

A few reformers in academic medicine sought to manage actively the application of advancing science to community medical practice. Between 1910 and the early 1920s, Ernest Codman had irritated colleagues in elite medicine in Boston by devising ways to quantify the "end results" of particular surgeons operating in particular hospitals.[18] In the mid-1930s, John Paul, a professor of medicine at Yale, proposed to use epidemiological methods to evaluate practice in order to improve it.[19] Hugh Cabot, who served as professor of surgery at Harvard, professor and dean at the University of Michigan and then chief surgeon of the Mayo Clinic, insisted in 1939 that the "individual physician is no longer in a position to come to safe judgments without conferring with his colleagues" organized in a hierarchy of expertise.[20]

THE POLITICS OF RESEARCH ON HEALTH SERVICES IN BRITAIN

As I described in Chapter 1, British leadership in devising and applying methods for studying events in populations, and particularly the effectiveness of interventions, made an essential contribution to the convergence of research and policymaking in the United States. During the interwar years, British researchers made significant innovations in the methodology of randomized controlled trials (RCTs), despite the unwillingness of the publicly financed Medical Research Council, according to a recent study, "to adopt statistical design in its clinical trials of the 1930s."[21]

Moreover, many researchers in Britain who studied the broad determinants of health and the natural history of disease had, since the mid-nineteenth century, also evaluated the effectiveness of health services and participated in policymaking for health. William Farr, a physician who served as chief statistician for the Office of the Register General is a notable example.[22] What came to be called "social medicine" worldwide during the 1920s and 1930s had considerably more legitimacy and influence on policy in Britain than in the United States.[23]

British researchers worked in a different political context from their American counterparts. Britain had enacted a limited program of national health insurance in 1911. After World War I, the central government and local authorities subsidized voluntary hospitals and built or renovated public hospitals to serve the middle class as well as the poor. In preparation for World War II, the government temporarily nationalized most hospitals and paid salaries to the physicians and surgeous who staffed them. The wartime coalition government announced in 1941 that a national hospital system would be established after the war. In 1943, public officials, consulting with leaders of the medical profession, began to plan a postwar health service.[24]

Between 1943 and 1945, intense debate occurred about many aspects of what became the National Health Service (NHS) in legislation enacted in 1946. But there was also widespread agreement that universal coverage was essential and imminent, that it should be financed predominantly by the public sector, and that services should be organized to facilitate the dissemination of scientific advances from teaching hospitals to general hospitals and from academics to consultants (called specialists in the United States) and general practitioners.

Unlike their American counterparts, researchers who studied health services in Britain participated in a consensus on policy reform. As a result they could, without fear of reprisal, engage in objective scientific research, conduct public advocacy on behalf of particular policy, and serve as formal advisers to policymakers. Moreover, their research, advocacy, and advice could include both improving health services and addressing broad socioeconomic determinants of health. In sharp contrast, even into the 1950s, medical and pharmaceutical interest groups in the United States often attacked the reputations and jobs of researchers, however objective their publications, who advocated (or sometimes merely seemed to advocate) reform either publicly or as employees of government.

This consensus in Britain sustained agreement about the scope of research to support the NHS. Maintaining an effective and efficient national service would require policymakers and managers to understand the health status of the population as well as what threatened and improved it. Because the NHS was funded entirely from tax revenue, it would be prudent policy to evaluate the influence of every potential determinant of health; including socioeconomic and cultural factors, nutrition, and individual behavior, as well as public and personal health services. Questions about the cost and organization of care should also be addressed within an intellectual framework that included population health.

Richard Titmuss, who in the early 1950s was principal investigator for the first national study of the cost of the NHS, exemplified the British consensus about the scope of research on health and health services. Titmuss began his career conducting studies of fertility. He evaluated the effects of broad social policy during the war on the health, economic status, and morale of the population of Britain in a landmark book published in 1950.[25] Brian Abel Smith, an economist who collaborated with Titmuss on the cost study, went on to an eminent career of policy advising, advocacy, and research on the cost-effectiveness and organization of health services.[26]

Archie Cochrane similarly exemplified the British consensus on the scope of research. As an undergraduate at Cambridge, Cochrane did laboratory research on tissue culture. In medical school at University College Hospital in London, he encountered Sir Thomas Lewis, a pioneer in research on heart disease that combined animal studies with research on patients. He also interrupted his studies to fight for the Loyalist cause in the Spanish Civil War. As an epidemiologist, Cochrane mainly studied the course of diseases of the lungs, especially among coal miners in Wales. But he also evaluated interventions and encouraged the young science of research synthesis. The Cochrane Collaboration, established and named after his death, became the world's leading organization in setting standards for and producing systematic reviews of health services.[27]

Many British epidemiologists, statisticians, and other participants in social medicine complained in the 1930s and 1940s that most clinicians valued research in the basic and clinical sciences more highly than their work. Nevertheless, until recently (as I describe in Chapter 5), government and foundations in Britain have subsidized research on health status and health services relatively more generously than funders in the United States. A recent assessment of British research on health in these years concluded that "epidemiology with its focus on whole populations had a ready political acceptance and its results had some chance of influencing policy."[28] Social medicine, although marginal in both countries, was considerably less marginal in Britain.

Most American epidemiologists and other researchers on health services, even those associated with social medicine, found it prudent to avoid addressing, in public at least, problems of the organization, financing, and utilization of health services. Frank Boudreau, an epidemiologist who became internationally prominent in social medicine as an official of the League of Nations Health Organization, typified his generation. The Milbank Memorial Fund appointed Boudreau as its chief executive in 1937 to repair the damage to its reputation as a result of the attacks by organized medicine on John Kingsbury's program. For the next two decades, Boudreau promoted a politically neutral, sometimes even apolitical, approach to social medicine in the Fund's work on family planning, nutrition, and mental health.[29]

Another example of prudent silence among American epidemiologists, especially those employed by public agencies, was the reluctance of most of them to study chronic degenerative disease, even the relatively neutral subject of its incidence and prevalence, until the late 1940s. A significant reason for their reticence was that most physicians, wary of intrusion into their autonomous practice, defined chronic disease as a personal matter between patients and doctors. They wanted the authority of public health agencies limited to communicable diseases. In the early 1930s, for instance, soon after the chief statistician at Metropolitan Life declared that cancer was epidemic, all but three respondents to a survey of the chief health officers of American states and Canadian provinces said "they were doing nothing about adult hygiene or chronic disease."[30]

The few exceptions to the prudent silence of most researchers on health services were evaluations of the effects of interventions in infectious disease. Several historians have documented the uneasy relationship among state public health officials, elite specialists, and general practitioners in the dissemination and promotion of pneumococcal serotherapy in the 1920s and 1930s.[31] Another early example of evaluation in the United States was research by the New York Academy of Medicine in the early 1930s that found that the rate of maternal deaths in childbirth was rising as a result of physicians' "operative interference" and "incapacity in judgment." Despite objections from many physicians and organizations that represented them, these findings received considerable publicity and led to the establishment of committees to review maternal deaths in many cities.[32]

The evaluation of streptomycin exemplifies the contrasting political contexts of research on health services in the United States and Britain. In September 1945, researchers at the Mayo Clinic reported "that streptomycin showed promise in treating advanced cases of tuberculosis." This report generated widespread demand for the drug. The Veterans Administration (VA) and the PHS soon organized clinical trials to test its effectiveness. The VA researchers abandoned randomized controls amid internal controversy. The PHS study randomized.[33]

Almost simultaneously, the Medical Research Council of the United Kingdom launched a study its historian describes as the "first clinical trial to fully meet the requirements of sound methodological design." He ascribes the clarity of British research policy in this instance to the desire of policymakers to avoid a "free market" in streptomycin because it would be inequitable and thus violate the fundamental principle of the NHS. The trial, he writes, was "unfolding within a domestic drama, whose leading players were the MRC, the M[inistry] o[f] H[ealth], the British medical profession and the emerging NHS."[34]

Only a few years later, other investigators at the Mayo Clinic held a press conference to announce that treatment with a new drug, cortisone, caused the remission of symptoms of rheumatoid arthritis in a small trial conducted without a control group. The lead investigator, accompanied by the surgeon general of the United States, showed a film about the "miracle of cortisone" to members of Congress. NIH officials, at the request of the White House, conducted a global search for a botanical substitute for the cortical steroid that was the source of cortisone. They also asked Congress to create a National Institute of Arthritis that would demonstrate that the methods devised to conquer infectious disease would lead to triumph over chronic disease.

In 1951, in contrast, British researchers began an RCT of cortisone; the study, published in 1954, found that it was about as effective as aspirin in treating rheumatoid arthritis. However, the award of a Nobel Prize in 1950 to the researchers who discovered cortisone suggests that dominant scientific opinion worldwide had yet to embrace statistical methods for evaluating health services.[35] Social medicine, in most countries, remained subordinate to the alliance of basic scientists and clinicians who did research on pathophysiology in prestige, funding, and influence on policy for health research and services.

HEALTH SERVICES RESEARCH AND THE POLITICS OF AN EXPANDING HEALTH SECTOR, 1945–1975

Demand for research on health services that could inform policy in the United States because it was detached from the politics of reform increased after World War II. Organizations that wanted this research included agencies at all levels of government, hospital and medical associations, foundations, labor unions, integrated delivery systems (then called pre-paid group practices), and even pharmaceutical manufacturers.[36]

Increasing public spending for health services fueled much of this demand. State and metropolitan hospital planning agencies mandated by the Hill-Burton Act hired economists and statisticians. Economists in the federal government adapted methodology devised during and after the war to study the general economy in order to report on national expenditures for health services.

Associations of providers, professionals, and manufacturers employed researchers to analyze information pertinent to their members. At the end of the war, for example, the American Hospital Association established the Hospital [later Health] Research and Education Trust (HRET) to evaluate existing facilities and assess future needs. The AMA, Association of American Medical Colleges, and the predecessor of what is now the Blue Cross and Blue Shield Association (BCBSA)increased their internal capacity to do research. Pharmaceutical and chemical manufacturers established the Health Information Foundation in 1950 and in 1952 hired an academic sociologist, Odin Anderson, as its research director.

A few endowed foundations funded research on health services. The Commonwealth Fund and the Kellogg Foundation, for example, helped to finance HRET. Commonwealth sponsored a major study of medical education. The Milbank Memorial Fund commissioned research that contributed to policy for deinstitutionalizing persons with mental illness.[37]

Labor unions used research on health services to inform their new role in health insurance. Most unions negotiated about coverage provided by employers. Unions whose members had multiple employers, notably unions representing the construction trades and longshoremen, purchased insurance policies to which employers contributed. The United Mine Workers (UMW) purchased insurance with royalties on each ton of coal extracted. Many unions hired researchers as staff and consultants. The UMW employed public health physicians who conducted research on its members' health and health services.[38] John Dunlop, a Harvard economist who became secretary of labor in the Ford Administration, recalled that his "interest in medical care began in the early 1950s when I found myself [as a consultant to a union during collective bargaining] . . . in a position of having to propose whether to spend $250,000,000 of the railroad's money on health and welfare programs."[39]

Internal research capacity helped the new prepaid group practices attract subscribers and respond to criticism of the quality of their care from local medical societies. Physicians and managers at Kaiser Permanente on the West Coast and the Health Insurance Plan in New York City established research groups that achieved national recognition by the 1960s. The labor unions on which both organizations depended heavily for subscribers valued their investment in research.

Most research on health services, however, addressed issues of access, supply, and cost rather than quality and effectiveness until the 1970s. Researchers, as well as their sponsors and employers, accorded priority to assessing the adequacy of the supply of hospitals, clinics, and health professionals and barriers to the utilization of services. Some sponsors encouraged researchers to explore the cultural context of illness—for example, in studies that, as the medical sociologist Samuel Bloom explained, "joined social science and psychiatry."[40]

A few academics challenged the priorities of this research. In 1950, for instance, Eli Ginzberg, a labor economist at Columbia University, called attention to broad determinants of health at the first session devoted to health economics in the history of the American Economic Association. Ginzberg challenged the assumption that there was a causal relationship between "striking advances" in biomedical science and population health. Despite the withdrawal of 40 percent of physicians from civilian practice, he said, the health of Americans with low incomes had improved during World War II.[41]

Other researchers sought to improve the effectiveness and efficiency of organizations that delivered health services. Walter McNerny of the University of Michigan and later the BCBSA evaluated the performance of hospitals. John D. Thompson of Yale, who studied the allocation of resources within hospitals, used and improved epidemiological methods introduced in Britain by Florence Nightingale in the nineteenth century. A growing number of academic physicians encouraged research on the effectiveness of primary and specialty care in ambulatory settings, notably Osler L. Peterson at North Carolina and Kerr White also at North Carolina and then Hopkins. A few investigators devised methods to measure and improve the quality of care by individual physicians, for example, Avedis Donabedian at the University of Michigan. Others evaluated the performance of large health plans, for example, Paul Denson and Sam Shapiro at the Health Insurance Plan of New York.

The postwar expansion of higher education for the health professions increased opportunities to conduct research on health services and train a new generation of investigators. Academic institutions were preparing a growing number of students for an expanding array of professions. Many of these students acquired their clinical skills in new or newly enlarged hospitals and clinics that academic institutions owned or dominated. Universities' research budgets increased, mainly as a result of the rapid growth of the extramural research program of the National Institutes of Health, but also because the federal government was, for the first time, awarding grants and contracts for research on health services.

The growing number of academics who studied health services reinforced disassociation between research and reform. This disassociation had begun in the 1930s and increased during the 1940s as a tactical response to attacks by organized medicine. Now it became a matter of principle. Criteria for appointment to and promotion and tenure in faculty positions rewarded research and teaching that sought to be both objective and neutral about policy and politics. Academics also had more freedom to select research questions and address them in depth than their colleagues who were employed by government, trade, and professional associations, provider organizations, industry-funded research centers, and foundations. As a result, fewer journal articles that reported the results of research on health services blended research and advocacy. An increasing number of articles in journals of health services research emphasized methodological and theoretical issues and accorded modest attention to policy and practice.

Researchers at every stage of their careers benefited from the expansion of higher education for the health professions. Odin Anderson moved the Health Information Foundation to the University of Chicago in 1962. Other established researchers like Denson, Shapiro, the economist Herbert Klarman, and the sociologist Raymond Fink moved to professorships (at Harvard, Hopkins, New York University, and New York Medical College, respectively) from jobs in planning organizations, labor unions, and prepaid group practices. Newly trained researchers, both Ph.D.s and health professionals, frequently had several job offers.

The establishment of a new institution, the academic health center (AHC), during the 1950s and 1960s, facilitated expansion of the field that had begun to be called health services research by 1960. AHCs integrated under a single university official responsibility for educating health professionals and managing the hospitals and clinics owned or affiliated with universities. Generous appropriations by state government enabled AHCs, almost two-thirds of which were public institutions, to hire new faculty from every discipline that studied health services and for a time to subsidize some of their research.[42]

Many chief executives of AHCs encouraged research on health services. Several of them had commissioned research on health services as public officials or managers in health care organizations; for example, Cecil G. Sheps at the University of North Carolina, and Philip R. Lee at the University of California, San Francisco, both of whom had also been co-investigators.

Moreover, many state officials and a few influential academic physicians wanted AHCs to become the dominant provider organizations as well as educational institutions in their geographic regions. Research was a source of useful information about AHCs' regions; for example about the distribution and cost of services and its relationship to the burden of disease. AHC chief executives allocated funds for deans and department chairs to hire social scientists and physicians trained in public health and research on health services. AHCs that did not have schools of public health established departments of community medicine. Demand for faculty was so great that some newly hired social scientists had never done research on health services.

The Clinical Scholars Program, conducted at leading AHCs since 1969, has trained several generations of physicians who have just completed their specialty training in the methods of health services research, and particularly in using them to evaluate the effectiveness of care. The Commonwealth Fund and the Carnegie Corporation funded the program until 1972. The Robert Wood Johnson Foundation has sponsored it since 1972. Many former Clinical Scholars became leaders in the field.

Institutions that were not public AHCs or even AHCs at all also contributed to the growing prestige of research on health services. The University of Pennsylvania established the Leonard Davis Institute of Health Economics in 1967. John Dunlop and Robert Ebert established an interfaculty program in health policy. Ebert, an internist who promoted prepaid group practice, had become dean of the Harvard Medical School in 1964.

Dunlop and Ebert wanted to link research in clinical epidemiology with economic analysis. Dunlop had an unusually broad definition of the economics of human resources. Ebert had followed British science, including research evaluating health services and the health of populations, since the late 1930s when, as a Rhodes Scholar, he participated in the initial research on the use of penicillin.

An opportunity to demonstrate the linkage of epidemiology and economics occurred in 1965 when a committee of the federal Bureau of the Budget (BoB, which was renamed the Office of Management and Budget) appointed Gerald Rosenthal to a committee charged to study the effectiveness and cost-effectiveness of different treatments for End-Stage Renal Disease (ESRD). Rosenthal, a faculty member at Harvard and then Brandeis University, had been a student of Dunlop's and a participant in the interfaculty seminar. HRET had published his doctoral dissertation on the demand for hospital services. Rosenthal and Herbert Klarman conducted a cost-effectiveness analysis for the BoB committee that subsequently influenced an amendment to the Social Security Act (in 1972) to extend Medicare coverage for ESRD to persons of all ages.[43]

Leaders of some prominent organizations of the health sector wanted medical schools and AHCs to remedy deficiencies in the quality of care that researchers had begun to document in the 1950s. State officials wanted health planning agencies mandated by the Hill-Burton Act and AHCs to improve quality by assuring that each region had the appropriate complement of specialized physicians and hospitals. They also expected alumni of AHC schools to improve quality in every health profession.

Dominant regional payers for private health insurance, especially Blue Cross and Blue Shield plans, shared state officials' desire for AHCs to improve the quality of health services. Executives of Blue plans and state officials collaborated on reimbursement policy, for example, to privilege academic centers at the expense of small, and especially proprietary, hospitals. In New York State, the collaboration was so close that the dominant Blue plan and the state's Department of Health became co-regulators of health-care facilities and financing.[44]

State officials and insurance executives overestimated the ability of AHCs to influence the medical profession. Intraprofessional politics during the first four decades of the century had resulted in a tacit, often begrudging, but effective division of authority within the profession. The division of authority led to its fragmentation.

The AMA, allied with state and county medical societies, had worked to divide authority since the 1920s in order to weaken or neutralize reformers who advocated the creation of hierarchies of specialized physicians and hospitals in geographic regions. Leaders of organized medicine lobbied governors and legislators to protect the long-standing dominance of community physicians on the public boards that licensed physicians and disciplined those who harmed or endangered patients. Local physicians also controlled the medical staff organizations of community hospitals. These organizations, rubber-stamped by hospital boards of trustees, awarded hospital "privileges" to physicians. Secure in its control of licensing and privileging, organized medicine usually acknowledged the dominance of academic physicians in policy for undergraduate medical education, residency and postresidency training, and in deciding which community physicians could admit patients to teaching hospitals.[45]

The division of authority was nuanced. Organized medicine had a formal role in accrediting medical schools. The AMA joined associations of academics in lobbying for increased funding for biomedical research. Academics were occasionally appointed to state licensing boards and often influenced the policy of the nonprofit boards that certified specialists and subspecialists.

Academics no longer dominated the growth of specialization, as they had in the late nineteenth and early twentieth centuries. A historian of specialization concluded in 2006 that, in the United States, in contrast to Britain, "medical domination of specialty training took place in a uniquely decentralized medical context in which power of all sorts was highly fragmented."[46]

The fragmentation of authority influenced how researchers evaluated the work of physicians. The first generation of researchers on what almost everyone in medicine called quality (a euphemism for reducing the incidence of poor care) had no practical alternative to accepting that physicians' authority to license, certify, and accord hospital privileges gave them exclusive control of measuring and evaluating clinicians' work and, when necessary, improving its quality. Researchers who studied quality encountered considerable resistance. Evidence of variation in the use of particular interventions and the effectiveness of physicians' work was also evidence of the effects of divided authority. Because public officials and insurance executives accepted divided authority, most physicians ignored evidence of variation and inferior practice until, in the 1980s, it began to be inescapable.

Researchers were just one of the groups resented by physicians, academics as well as community practitioners, for intruding into their clinical autonomy. These groups included anti-trust regulators (who challenged physicians' monopoly of fees, referrals, and the organization of practice), state attorneys general (who investigated fraudulent use of public reimbursement), the medical staff of public and private payers (who made decisions about what services were "medically necessary") and, above all, lawyers for plaintiffs in litigation about malpractice.

The main causes of intrusion from all sources were increasing expenditures for health care by the federal and state government and private employers and the introduction of new technologies. Physicians found it difficult to address the drivers of cost described in Chapter 1, especially the proliferation and often misuse of technologies that contributed to professional satisfaction and rising incomes.

Leading researchers tried to accommodate the methodology for assessing quality in order to improve it to the divided, but nevertheless comprehensive, authority of physicians over the profession's practice. Avedis Donabedian, for example, published a seminal paper on evaluating quality in 1966. He distinguished his recommendations for measuring the process, structure, and outcomes of care from the "value judgments" of elite clinicians in the past.[47] Researchers working for the CCMC had collected and summarized these value judgments. The majority of CCMC members had used them to justify organizing physicians in hierarchies of multi-specialty groups paid by government and insurance companies. Donabedian relied heavily on a paper by Mindel C. Sheps published a decade earlier. Sheps had described the CCMC's standards for quality as having been "derived empirically," a euphemism for the opinions of elite physicians.[48] What she and then Donabedian proposed would eventually become even more threatening to physicians' autonomy: formal measurement of their behavior and its effects on patients' health.

This threat became evident to some people in the health sector in the 1970s when John Wennberg began to document variation in medical practice among regions and smaller geographic areas that was independent of the incidence and prevalence of disease—what came to be called unwarranted variation. In 1973, Wennberg and Alan Gittlesohn published a landmark study of variation in rates of tonsillectomies among small geographic areas of northern New England. Wennberg did not draw conclusions about the quality of care from his research. Neither did he comment publicly about the locus of responsibility for measuring quality and reducing unwarranted variation.[49] Lecturing on variation to physicians at an AHC in the mid-1970s, his opening sardonic words were, "I'm an epidemiologist; I don't have hypotheses." Wennberg understood the toxic legacy of the association of research on health services with reform.

The field of health services research was acquiring unprecedented legitimacy in the mid-1970s. The federal government had established a National

Center for Health Services Research and Development (NCHSR&D) in 1968 in order to consolidate and expand grant programs scattered among PHS agencies. More researchers studied health services than ever before. A growing number of researchers in both the social sciences and the health professions used statistical methods to study events in populations prospectively, including the effects and effectiveness of clinical interventions. The field had several dedicated journals. Moreover, major journals of the medical profession and its specialties now published occasional articles based on health services research. In 1974, Gerald Rosenthal became the first nonphysician director of the renamed NCHSR (Congress had removed "Development" from its title that year).

RESEARCH ON THE EFFECTIVENESS OF HEALTH SERVICES, 1975–1990

Federal funding for health services research was, however, in considerable jeopardy in 1975, the year Gerald Rosenthal announced that the "quality of care" would replace access to health services as the highest priority of NCHSR.[50] Members of the congressional staff had told Rosenthal that the research NCHSR sponsored lacked practical applications. Congress reduced its budget and eliminated its program of grants for research training, most of which had been awarded to AHCs.

Health services research had already become a lower priority for AHCs. Government in most states was reducing appropriations for them as a result of the oil crisis and "stagflation." Chief executives of AHCs and the deans and hospital directors who reported to them were preoccupied with maximizing revenue from clinical services and grants from NIH for research in the basic health sciences and its clinical applications.

Moreover, the medical staffs of community hospitals were resisting academic encroachment more effectively. They were able to do this because most of the residents and clinical fellows trained in AHCs chose to practice in community hospitals in regions surrounding them. The politics of health finance required government and insurance plans to reimburse the procedures they performed. AHCs now competed for patients who would have been referred to them a few years earlier.

AHC chief executives and medical school deans valued biomedical research funding more highly than ever before. More money from NIH brought higher institutional prestige, which made it easier to recruit faculty who would attract even more funding for research, graduate student stipends and post doctoral fellowships. As a result of the perpetual budget crisis that began in the mid-1970s, moreover, AHC leaders became increasingly dependent on the generous overhead that accompanied grants from NIH.

AHC chief executives no longer had incentives to insulate health services researchers from the consequences of the low value accorded their work by most of their colleagues in the basic science and clinical disciplines. Without protection from AHC leadership, many health services researchers struggled to maintain the percentage of their salaries paid in hard money and to retain teaching hours in the curricula of schools of the health professions. Institutional subsidies for research on health services vanished.

Internal conflict prevented the field of health services research from presenting a unified case for greater recognition during the 1970s. Many researchers resented Rosenthal's changes in the organization and priorities of NCHSR. Some of them complained because the number and size of its investigator-initiated grants declined when Rosenthal reallocated funds to targeted intramural and commissioned research that was designed to be useful to policymakers.

Other researchers attacked NCHSR's new priority of quality as a betrayal of reform that would expand access to care. Many medical sociologists criticized a talk by an associate director of NCHSR about its new priorities at a meeting of their section of the American Sociological Association in 1976. Some of them said they resented the priority accorded to quality because they studied access; others that achieving universal coverage should be the highest priority of researchers. Several participants accused Rosenthal of deemphasizing research on access because, as an economist, he had an ideological preference for market-based rather than public policy solutions to problems of health services. A few said that they resented the growing influence of economists on health policy.

Such internal conflict prevented the formation of a national organization to represent the field, especially to Congress, until the early 1980s. Most health services researchers continued to identify mainly with organizations that represented their clinical, public health, or social science disciplines.

Rosenthal and his senior staff sought new supporters for NCHSR and hence for the field. They sought advice about the agency's priorities and projects from officers and staff of leaders of the "House of Medicine," that is, of organizations that accredited medical schools, and examined, licensed, certified, and lobbied on behalf of physicians. One result of this effort was that NCHSR staff and colleagues in the Bureau of Health Manpower convened nineteen senior health professionals in the "first [group] to address the relationship between research on professional education and public policy." The group finessed divided authority in medicine with the empirical observation that "professional education has largely been a different world from professional practice."[51]

NCHSR also sought to inform state policymakers about the methods and uses of research on health services. Soon after announcing that quality was its highest priority, the agency created a User Liaison Program (ULP) to inform state legislators and officials of the executive branch. Robert A. Fordham, a career federal civil servant, organized this work. Fordham had become familiar with health service research as special assistant to Philip R. Lee, assistant secretary for health in the Johnson Administration. While on temporary assignment as a dean at the University of Vermont in the early 1970s, he had worked with legislators and policymakers in the executive branch. He met Wennberg and learned about his research in northern New England. Fordham was also intrigued by the potential uses of research by Lawrence Weed, a faculty member at the University of Vermont, who was redesigning the medical record in order to improve the quality of care. Fordham left Vermont late in 1974 to become special assistant to Rosenthal.

The ULP convened interactive workshops of 30–40 state officials and 7–10 researchers to discuss research relevant to an issue in health policy. Beginning in 1979, the ULP also conducted longer workshops to introduce policymakers to the methods and potential uses of the broad field of health services research.

Fordham used several techniques to maximize the influence of the workshops on policymakers. He discouraged them from leaving early and being distracted by events in their home states by convening meetings at remote conference centers that provided few public telephones. Timberline Lodge on Mt. Hood became a favorite site because it was ninety minutes from the nearest international airport and its postal address, Government Camp, immunized elected officials against accusations that they had been on a junket. Participants in ULP meetings sat in a hollow square. Presentations by researchers were brief; considerable time was left for discussion. Fordham excluded the officials' staff or any other observers. He encouraged officials to attend as many meetings as they could and pressed them to recommend colleagues.

The ULP was a new way to inform policymakers about research. Researchers typically disseminated their findings by publishing articles in scientific journals. Their findings also reached policymakers and their staff in occasional press accounts of their work, through their participation in committees that wrote reports or advised public officials, and, occasionally, in testimony before legislative committees.

Fordham asked state officials to help him plan workshops and to criticize the presentations of researchers at rehearsals for them. He also pressed the participants in each meeting to submit anonymous reports evaluating each of the presentations and the discussion following them. Then he sent the scores of and comments about each researcher to every researcher who participated.

Fordham acquired a constituency of state officials who responded promptly and effectively to his occasional requests for them to intervene with members of Congress in support of the budget of the ULP. Moreover, as a senior NCHSR official who resented Fordham's independence complained to a former federal colleague, the members of Congress from Vermont represented the ULP as well as the state.

EVALUATING THE EFFECTIVENESS OF HEALTH SERVICES, 1975–2000

Research on the effectiveness and efficiency of health services became increasingly important to policymakers in the public and private sectors over the next quarter century. Slowing the rate of growth in spending while maintaining the quality of care was the highest priority of most of them; next came expanding access when funds permitted.

John Wennberg's research, which now examined evidence of variation across the country, continued to suggest that considerable care might be inappropriate and hence wasteful and perhaps harmful. In an article in 1984, he argued that documenting and assessing the causes of unwarranted variation could be the basis for policy to improve the effectiveness and efficiency of care. He invited policymakers and physicians to test the proposition that "feedback of information on practice variations and outcomes . . . will result in the reconsideration [by physicians] of the indicators for specific services." Wennberg hoped that physicians' assessment of the reasons for variation would motivate them to base their recommendations to patients on higher standards of evidence. After physicians were properly informed about practice variations and outcomes, he wrote, "Some [remaining] controversies concerning the need for or value of specific practices will be resolved through a critical review of the medical literature or by the application of decision analysis."[52]

Most British researchers on health services, in contrast, believed that producing better evidence about the effectiveness of interventions was the precondition for raising physicians' standards of practice. During the 1980s, they advocated conducting more RCTs and systematic reviews of them.

Wennberg continued to rely on administrative data for his own research. He acknowledged British research on variation rather than on effectiveness. But he had a more comprehensive view of the field of health services research than many of his American colleagues. For example, he praised both the Clinical Scholars program, which trained researchers mainly in the methods of observational research, and the Milbank Fellows program, which sent young physicians to Britain to study prospective research in clinical epidemiology.

Most American researchers shared Wennberg's preference for conducting rigorous observational research using administrative data. They argued that their research promised useful results in less time and at lower cost than most of the RCTs conducted in the United States. Leading observational researchers included Paul Ellwood (Interstudy), John Bunker (Stanford University), David Eddy (Duke University and the AMA), Robert Brook (the RAND Corporation and the University of California at Los Angeles), Donald Berwick (Harvard), and Sheldon Greenfield (UCLA and Tufts).

Two characteristics of most RCTs conducted in the United States justified their preference for observational research. One, as described in Chapter 1, was that pharmaceutical companies financed most RCTs under contracts with academic medical centers and, increasingly, with private companies that frequently restricted investigators' intellectual freedom. Since the 1930s, according to a historian of "rational medical practice," RCTs had become the "standard of proof for new therapies." But they were not the standard for evaluating established interventions in the United States.[53]

The second objection was that RCTs were inefficient. Most American RCTs, in contrast to large trials in other countries, enrolled patients being treated in teaching hospitals and their clinics. Critics complained that these RCTs evaluated interventions under ideal conditions (which they called efficacy) rather than in the ordinary practice of medicine (described as effectiveness). Moreover, this research was expensive, time-consuming, had low priority for federal funding, and raised ethical questions if some patients did not receive a potentially effective treatment or could not be properly randomized.

RCTs conducted in other industrial countries, in contrast, frequently enrolled large numbers of patients being treated in ordinary community practices. In the United States, community trials began to receive substantial funding only in the late 1980s, as NIH responded to demand for them from advocates for persons with AIDS/HIV and their supporters among researchers.[54]

A growing number of American researchers, however, were conducting RCTs and following the development of the methodology of systematic reviews by their colleagues in other countries. Members of this group included Suzanne and Robert Fletcher (University of North Carolina, American College of Physicians and Harvard), Thomas Chalmers (Mount Sinai School of Medicine and Harvard), and Frederick Mosteller (Harvard). Alvin Feinstein (Yale) was a sharp critic of the methodology of RCTs and systematic reviews but shared the interest of their defenders in using advanced statistical methods to improve clinical judgment.[55]

Americans also differed from colleagues in other industrial countries in how they used the methodology of technology assessment (TA). TA developed in the 1960s mainly among American scientists and engineers who were concerned about unanticipated consequences of industrial and agricultural processes. The name was first used in a 1965 report by the Committee on Science and Astronautics of the U.S. House of Representatives. In 1969, Congress commissioned an assessment of new health screening technology from the National Academy of Engineering. Three years later it created an Office of Technology Assessment (OTA). In 1975 NCHSR hired a staff member, Sherry Arnstein, who was co-author of a new book, *Perspectives on Technology Assessment*.[56] OTA issued an influential report on CT scanning, an imaging technology, in 1978. The same year Congress created a National Center for Health Care Technology Assessment (NCHCTA).[57]

TA threatened the interests of manufacturers of medical devices and pharmaceutical drugs. The questions asked in assessments were considerably broader, especially about clinical and environmental effects, than those manufacturers had to answer to obtain federal approval to bring products to market. Moreover assessments frequently compared competing technologies. Manufacturers and their allies persuaded Congress to abolish NCHCTA early in the Reagan administration. Proponents of TA among provider organizations, large purchasers, and health professionals tried to replace it with a series of public/private programs but failed to mobilize sufficient support to sustain them.

Because of this history, the organizations that have conducted a considerable amount of health TA in the United States since the 1980s did not receive public funding for it. Most of them financed TA by selling subscriptions to their reports to hospitals and health plans. They also competed for contracts to assist agencies of the federal government in making decisions about technology. Leading organizations using this business model included the ECRI Institute (founded as the Emergency Care Research Institute), Battelle Memorial Institute, and the BCBSA Technology Evaluation Center (TEC).

The TA business model usually precluded publication of findings from assessments in peer-reviewed journals in order to preserve their cash value to subscribing organizations. Because the journals that academics read did not publish articles based on TAs, most academic researchers did not follow the development of its methodology or learn the results of its application. The executives who purchased medical equipment for hospitals did not routinely share more than summaries of the TA they subscribed to with physicians; almost all of whom, moreover, received biased TA from manufacturers. The media reported on assessments only in the course of investigating provider organizations for conflict of interest, self-dealing, or fraudulent procurement practices.

The history of TA has been different in other industrial countries. Since the 1980s, in Australia, Canada, New Zealand, the Netherlands, the Nordic Countries and the United Kingdom, for example, government subsidized TA and encouraged publication of assessments. TA became one among a variety of methods with which persons who conducted and consumed research on health services were familiar. Because TA integrated work in a variety of disciplines, the phrase gradually became a synonym for the broad field of research on the effectiveness and efficiency of health services.[58]

A similar integration of TA with RCTs, systematic reviews, observational research, and cost-effectiveness analysis began to occur in the United States during the late 1990s. But most people who follow research in the health sector still define it as the evaluation of medical devices and equipment. A considerable amount of sophisticated TA is, moreover, still financed by subscription and not published in peer-reviewed journals or free-standing reports or posted on Web sites. Provider organizations and health plans frequently use the results of TA they commission, conduct, or subscribe to in order to seek a competitive advantage.

Despite differences between the United States and other industrial countries in the financing and coordination of research on health services,

American policymakers have made increasing use of its findings during the past quarter century. A signal event occurred in 1986 when the federal Health Care Financing Agency (HCFA, now the Centers for Medicare and Medicaid Services, or CMS) began to publish data comparing risk adjusted rates of death among Medicare beneficiaries in hospitals. Measuring and improving quality had become a high priority for HCFA after 1983, when Congress enacted the Prospective Payment System (PPS) for paying hospitals. Under PPS hospitals received a single payment for each episode of hospitalization, calculated in units called Disease Related Groups (DRGs). DRGs were based on research by John D. Thompson and Robert Fetter that NCHSR had funded. Hospitals now had an incentive to discharge patients "sicker and quicker," in a phrase widely used at the time. To reduce this incentive, HCFA, under Administrator William Roper (1986–89), began to compare and report on mortality among hospitals. These reports attracted considerable attention in the media.

Many physicians, even in highly rated hospitals, condemned this intrusion on their autonomy. At a public sector academic health center that still sought to have some regional influence, for example, the office of its chief executive commissioned economists at the university to adapt the HCFA methodology in order to compare mortality in populations not covered by Medicare at the approximately twenty hospitals that served the three million people of the region. The state's department of health released the data required to conduct the study. The medical board of the AHC's teaching hospital opposed the study as intrusive. The chief executive cancelled it.

Despite such resistance, Roper recommended more intrusion. In an article in the *New England Journal of Medicine* in 1988 he and colleagues proposed "an initiative to evaluate and improve medical practice." Moreover, he substituted the phrase "effectiveness in health care" for the euphemistic "quality," defining effectiveness as both "efficiency" and "appropriateness." The authors acknowledged that the "science of health care evaluation . . . is still in its infancy," but they cited notable examples of research by Americans.[59]

With strong support from Roper and the White House, Congress in 1989 renamed NCHSR the Agency for Health Care Policy and Research (AHCPR) and charged it to improve effectiveness. A historian of AHCPR concluded that its creation and funding exemplified acceptance of the "idea that the federal government should allocate significant resources to researching the outcomes and effectiveness of medical procedures." AHCPR's budget nearly doubled over the next several years.[60]

In the early 1990s, health services research seemed to be appropriately organized and sufficiently well financed to inform policy. Gail Wilensky, who succeeded Roper as HCFA administrator, was a health economist and had worked in the intramural research program at NCHSR. Carl Schramm, who had conducted research on financing health services as a faculty member at Johns Hopkins, became chief executive of the Health Insurance Association of America (now America's Health Plans). Other health services researchers had recently been appointed as chief executives of national foundations; for instance, the Commonwealth Fund, the William T. Grant Foundation, the Kaiser Family Foundation, the Milbank Memorial Fund, and the Robert Wood Johnson Foundation.

In 1995, however, AHCPR "narrowly escaped being eliminated" as a result of the strongest attack on research on health services by physicians since organized medicine had rejected the work of the CCMC and the Milbank Memorial Fund sixty years earlier. Members of the new Republican majority in the House and Senate attempted to eliminate the agency because of its alleged interference with the practice of medicine and what its historian described as its general inefficiency. AHCPR had, he wrote, "committed enemies" in medicine as a result of its sponsorship of research on effectiveness and in particular of a clinical practice guideline it issued on surgery for low back pain. The agency was also tainted by its association with the failed Clinton health plan. Moreover, it still experienced the long-standing problem of health services research—having "too few friends" in influential positions in health affairs, politics, and the media.[61]

AHCPR survived because the field was acquiring such friends. The AMA House of Delegates and the Executive Board of the Association of American Medical Colleges passed resolutions of support. The Academy of Family Physicians testified to a committee of Congress on its behalf. Associations of hospitals, nurses and the health insurance industry told members of Congress that the agency should continue.

AHCPR was also expanding the scope of the methodology that it supported. In 1997, it designated Evidence Based Practice Centers (EPCs) in the United States and Canada to conduct systematic reviews, which it called "evidence reports," and technology assessments. The EPCs competed for funding to conduct reviews and assessments that AHCPR coordinated on behalf of HCFA and external organizations. Senior staff of AHCPR soon began to attend the International Cochrane Colloquium and participate in its Funders Forum. The U.S. Cochrane Center subsequently received several grants to encourage the production and enhance the quality of systematic reviews.

Organizations that provided and paid for health services to large populations were also spending more to evaluate health services. Like AHCPR, they accorded more attention to research methods that had been used with greater frequency by researchers in other countries. Within the federal government, the Health Care Financing Administration and the Department of Veterans Affairs raised the salience of research findings on effectiveness. Integrated delivery systems like Kaiser Permanente, the Group Health Cooperative of Puget Sound and Health Partners increased their capacity to conduct research and analysis. Managers of health benefits for a few Fortune 100 companies insisted that coverage decisions and standards for selecting providers be informed by research. Major insurance plans that administered benefits for these corporations increased their use of research findings.

RESEARCH ON EFFECTIVENESS AND THE STATES, 1999–2002

Reports by the Institute of Medicine (IOM) on safety (2000) and on quality (2001) raised the salience of these issues for public and private purchasers, providers and, as a result of extensive coverage in the media, for the public. The first report, *To Err Is Human*, estimated that between 44,000 and 98,000 deaths occurred each year as a result of errors in care in hospitals. The second, *Crossing the Quality Chasm*, documented unnecessary suffering and death as a result of unwarranted variation in medical practice and recommended ways to reduce it.[62]

Heightened concern about safety and quality stimulated new funding for research evaluating health services and more attention to findings from it. Appropriations for AHRQ grew. The Institute for Healthcare Improvement (IHI), led by Donald Berwick, used findings from research on effectiveness to inform the work of thousands of "collaboratives" of physicians and other health professionals. Conferences and publications proliferated.

Many clinical investigators, however, continued to accord low priority to research on effectiveness. In the summer of 2002, the *Journal of the American Medical Association* sent for peer review an article by nineteen leading researchers who comprised the IOM's Clinical Research Roundtable, "Central Challenges Facing the National Clinical Research Enterprise." The authors did not mention either research on effectiveness or the science of research synthesis and its principal product, systematic reviews. In the published article, however, the authors emphasized the importance of systematic reviews for policy and practice, appropriating verbatim language from one of the reviews.[63]

A significant number of senior policymakers in the states already understood the potential significance for policy of research on effectiveness and of systematic reviews in particular. Many state officials had been following the progress of this research at meetings convened by the ULP under Robert Fordham and his successors. Fordham had continued to convene meetings of state officials as a member of the staff of the Milbank Memorial Fund, which he joined in 1991. As a private operating foundation Milbank, unlike a federal agency, was not required to discourage state officials from discussing political issues in using the findings of research and making health policy.

In mid-2002, legislative leaders and senior executive branch officials from forty-two states, each of them a current or recent member of the Steering Committee of the Reforming States Group (RSG), submitted an article on policy for covering and purchasing prescription drugs to *Health Affairs*, a widely read journal of health policy. The officials documented the effects on state budgets of the rising cost of pharmaceutical drugs and recommended policy for solving the interrelated problems of drug coverage and costs. Their first recommendation was that states "look to researchers to supply evidence with immediate policy relevance, especially evidence from systematic review of medical literature, reviews produced, notably, by the Evidence-Based Practice Centers and the international Cochrane Collaboration."[64]

This chapter has described some of the events since the early twentieth century that made this recommendation possible. These events occurred at the intersection of the politics of organizing and financing health services with the methods of research on health services and the politics of the public and philanthropic organizations that sponsored such research.

The interrelationship of health politics and research on health services is, however, part of a more complicated story. What researchers did, how politics influenced what they studied, and the reception of their findings made possible the convergence that is the subject of this book. But what is possible frequently does not happen. The next chapter describes how legislators and officials of the executive branch in the states developed competencies that enabled them to appreciate and apply the findings of research on health services.

3. The Competence of States in Health Policy

Policymakers in the executive and legislative branches of state government have become increasingly adept at addressing the complexities of health politics and policy. Their expertise in health affairs prepared them to appreciate and use research evaluating the effectiveness of interventions.

Federalism is central to the story of the competence of state officials in health policy; but it is not the whole story. Federal funds, regulations and mandates have often been incentives for state officials to become more sophisticated public managers. Other incentives have, however, been independent of the federal government.

Political scientists and historians often describe three phases of federalism, but disagree about definitions and the duration of each phase. The Constitution created "dual federalism" in which the federal government and each of the states were sovereign entities. Dual federalism persisted, although disrupted by the Civil War and Reconstruction, until early in the twentieth century. "Cooperative" federalism," was the next phase, from the Progressive Era through the 1950s. During these years, the number and size of federal grants-in-aid to the states increased. Moreover, state policy sometimes preceded and influenced federal legislation; for example, old-age pensions and insurance against unemployment. But pervasive conflict about federal regulations, preemption, and unfunded mandates accompanied cooperation. The third phase, which some scholars call "coercive" and others "conflicted" federalism has since the 1960s been the source of considerable tension and conflict between the federal government and the states.[1]

Nobody I have worked with in state government during the past four decades has mentioned these abstractions. I suspect that if I asked my colleagues about them (which they would consider a strange request), many would describe their work as offering examples of dual, cooperative, and coercive federalism every day.

On the rare occasions when senior state officials talk abstractly about their work, they usually describe it as a struggle for scarce resources and authority. This struggle occurs within state government, between state and local government, and between the federal government and the states. The struggle almost always involves political partisanship, personal ambition, and the efforts of interest and advocacy groups to obtain more of whatever it is they seek.

GENERAL AND SPECIALIZED GOVERNMENT

The convergence that is the subject of this book occurred because elected officials and heads of executive branch agencies concluded that research findings could help them use their authority to spend scarce resources more effectively. After these policymakers became convinced that the methods of research evaluating services were persuasive and its results useful, they asked experts employed by state health agencies to devise processes through which the findings of research could inform policy for coverage. In some states, experts in these agencies had been aware of advances in health services research. But specialized civil servants do not have many opportunities to speak directly to elected and appointed officials, government generalists, on subjects of their own choosing.

The fundamental difference between generalists and specialists in state government is that generalists allocate while specialists advocate. Generalists distribute resources and authority among competing claimants within government as well as outside it. They include governors and legislators, their immediate staff, and persons whom governors appoint and legislators confirm to head agencies. General government often employs experts whose work includes being informed and skeptical about information and analysis offered to their bosses by experts in the line agencies of state government.

These agencies are specialized government. Unlike generalists, officials of specialized government are not obligated by constitutions and election cycles to care about which agencies other than their own win and lose in competing for resources or whether the residents of their state pay more or less in taxes and fees. Their priority is to justify, and advocate for, more money and authority for their agencies. Persons in specialized government are often, but not always, career officials. They often, but not always, have advanced education and training in a profession or an analytical discipline.

Generalists and specialists have considerable interaction. Specialists often justify the policy they recommend by citing findings from research. When these findings are weak or absent specialists usually ask generalists to trust their experience. They know that it is perilous to be caught distorting the information and analysis they present. However, they frequently encourage such distortion; for example, by asking interest and advocacy groups to lobby for appropriations to their agencies and on behalf of particular policies. Government generalists describe specialists who enlist lobbyists as disloyal.[2]

COMPETING PERCEPTIONS OF THE EFFECTIVENESS OF STATE GOVERNMENT

Disparagement of state government, both general and specialized, has a long history. Some scholars date it from the frustrations of governing under the Articles of Confederation that precipitated the Constitutional Convention in 1787. The modern version began during the Progressive Era of the early twentieth century. Much criticism of the capacity of states to govern since then has been based on the assumption that the expansion of centralized federal authority is an inevitable result of advances in technology, of the growth of interstate commerce and later a global economy, and of an increasingly mobile population. Other critics of state government have had narrower political agendas. Examples include advocates of civil rights who deplored "states' rights" as a euphemism for institutionalized racism; conservatives who complained that state taxation impeded economic growth; and liberals who argued that the persistence of states prevented the enactment of equitable health and social policy.[3]

Critics of states have, however, been flexible. Business executives have frequently complained about states' regulatory intrusion and lobbied the U.S. Congress to preempt state laws. Many of the same executives also pressed state government for tax write-offs, subsidized capital financing, and gifts of land by eminent domain. Advocates for universal health coverage have complained that states are "structural impediments" to national reform. But many of them have also described state initiatives to expand access to care as potential models for the nation. Proponents of economic growth through lower taxes and less intrusive regulation have, on other occasions, asked states to increase spending for education and highways. A reader of American history would be justified in concluding that states are "laboratories of democracy," in Justice Brandeis's famous phrase, except when they are not.[4]

Officials of local government routinely criticize state government. "Home rule," is a euphemism for the devolution of states' constitutional authority to levy taxes and determine the structure of local government. Disputes about home rule have occurred since the early nineteenth century. The most populous cities and counties have traditionally resisted, ignored and even defied state authority. New York City, for example, has never merged its vital statistics with those maintained by the state's department of health.

Officials of public universities frequently criticize the budgetary decisions of general government. They are more outspoken than most persons in specialized government because many of them do not self-identify as public employees. In 2005, for instance, the dean of a state's only medical school, complaining about declining appropriations, said that "this school used to be a public institution." The occasion was a lecture inaugurating a hall in the school's new building for which the state had subsidized capital financing. Several decades earlier, another frustrated medical dean had offered his stethoscope to a member of a governor's staff, saying: "Here, you take care of the patients."

Since the late nineteenth century, many academics and other experts on government have considered state government "dependent, subordinate and inferior," as Martha Derthick, a political scientist at the University of Virginia, wrote in 1996 and reprinted in 2001.[5] More than a century earlier, Simon N. Patten, an influential economist and teacher, had deplored the "decay" of state and local government, which, he said, was a result of their officials' increasing attention to national politics rather than to community interests.[6] Luther H. Gulick, a pioneer practitioner and scholar of what was then the new discipline of public administration, wrote in 1933 that states had become obsolete because they could not address the "life and death tasks of the new national economy."[7] In the mid-1980s, Wilbur Cohen, who had begun his long federal service early in the New Deal, recalled that Franklin Roosevelt "could have wiped out the states" in 1934–35 when they were "bankrupt sovereignties."[8] In 1971, John Gardner, who had been federal secretary of health, education and welfare, president of the Carnegie Corporation of New York and the first chief executive of the Urban Coalition, proclaimed that only a "mere handful" of states were "able to fulfill the . . . responsibilities inherent in the concept of federalism."[9] Alice Rivlin, an economist who has held several senior positions in the federal government, wrote in 1992 of the "escalating perception that states were performing badly even in areas that almost everyone regarded as properly assigned to them."[10]

Many experts, including those just quoted, also had more balanced opinions. Patten cherished memories of state government helping his legislator father and his neighbors develop the economy of DeKalb County, Illinois.[11] An admiring student of Patten's, Francis Perkins, was the strongest advocate of devolving authority to state government as secretary of labor in Franklin Roosevelt's cabinet.[12] Luther Gulick worked effectively with state officials as city administrator of New York in the mid-1950s. Wilbur Cohen was an architect of Medicaid as assistant secretary and then secretary of health, education and welfare under John F. Kennedy and Lyndon Johnson. John Gardner conceded that states had "vast residual responsibility." Rivlin proposed to "restructure" the responsibilities of the federal government and the states.

A few scholars have accorded states more prominent roles in contemporary history than most of their colleagues did. V. O. Key, a political scientist at Harvard, wrote in the mid-1950s that states were hardly "vestigial remnants." The "growth of federal power" and funding," he continued, had "liberate[d] the states" by making them less concerned about their "competitive position." Moreover, states had become more important than local government as sources of subsidy for roads, health and social services and, frequently, education. Key refused to consign American "nationhood" to the "finished professionals who operate in Washington."[13]

Similarly, Robert Wiebe of Northwestern University concluded that between the 1930s and 1950s, national and state leaders "traded support." In what he called the "compromise of the 1930s," leaders of the federal government "set broad economic policy." State officials and their allies in local government, business, unions and the professions "set the rules in their own localities, including how federal monies would be spent." Wiebe regretted that this compromise had broken down in the 1960s because of an "outpouring of national rules."[14]

Other scholars have described the resilience of state government despite the unprecedented assertion of federal authority that began in the 1960s. Daniel J. Elazar, a political scientist at Temple University, argued that states serve their citizens well because their policies reflect differences in political culture across the nation. As a result of these differences, "every state has certain dominant traditions about what constitutes proper government actions" and hence different policies and appetites for funding them.[15] Donald Kettl, a political scientist now at the University of Pennsylvania, observed in the mid-1980s that "nearly everything has become intergovernmental" rather than either federal or state.

Intergovernmentalism had "broadened participation in the crafting of federal policy" by creating a "specialized politics that operates at all levels of government."[16] Key, Wiebe, and Elazar respected the work of state officials in setting priorities and making policy in response to the demands of individuals and interest groups. Kettl, however, writing in 2002, accorded the theory of public administration and the academic analysis that underlies it higher "status" than the experience of state officials.[17]

Several scholars have recently demonstrated new respect for states' contribution to what William Novak in 2008 called the "infrastructural power" of government in the United States.[18] Chung Lae Cho and Deil Wright have adduced evidence that "states administrative capacities increased from the 1960s onward."[19] Kimberley S. Johnson found that the "ability of the national state to implement its policies" between 1877 and 1929 was "dependent on its ability to develop bureaucratic partners in the American states."[20] Andrew Karch, in a study of recent policy diffusion among American states, emphasized their "resurgence" to become a "main locus of policymaking" during the past generation.[21]

Most experts on state government in universities and research organizations have assumed that state officials have been preoccupied by relationships with federal agencies. This assumption has led them to focus their research on three periods of national reform; the Progressive Era (especially 1900–1917), what historians call the First New Deal (1933–36), and Lyndon Johnson's Great Society (1964–67). Summarizing the effects of these eras of reform on federalism, Derthick concluded, for instance, that states have become residual. They "retain a vitality born of the limits of national institutions' capacity." States have a role, she wrote, only when the federal government lacks "authority, revenue, will power, political consensus, [and] institutional capacity."[22]

Government in most states has, however, become increasingly competent at serving the needs of citizens. The competence of state government increased in part as a result of managing funds in federal grants and complying with federal regulations. But the competence of state government also increased as a result of its response to changes in the size, characteristics, location, sources of income, wealth and expectations of the American people. In health policy, states demonstrated competence in responding to changes in demography and public expectations years before the huge increase in federal funds and regulations that began in the late 1960s as a result of the enactment of Medicaid and Medicare.

STATES AND HEALTH POLICY

The competence of state government has steadily increased since 1787, when James Madison described their importance in the new "compound republic" of the United States.[23] Early state statutes established the responsibilities of local government for building and maintaining roads, aiding the sick and the poor, educating children, and protecting public safety. In response to growing population in rural areas as well as in cities in the early decades of the nineteenth century, states created agencies to build canals, roads, and bridges, to regulate commerce, and to collect data. Some of these agencies were corporations; precursors of the public benefit corporations that built and managed bridges, tunnels, world trade centers, and public teaching hospitals in the twentieth century.[24]

Policy to protect and, by the late nineteenth century, to improve health emerged from state officials' responsibility for stimulating and regulating the economy. Infectious disease inhibited manufacturing, agriculture, and commerce. In the first half of the nineteenth century, both of the competing theories of the causes of disease, environmental toxins (called miasmas) and germs, justified vigorous policy by state and local government to improve sanitation by constructing sewers, reservoirs and aqueducts. Each theory also justified quarantining travelers and isolating the sick during epidemics, especially the periodic outbreaks of yellow fever and cholera during the first half of the century. By the 1890s, germ theory was the basis of state and local health policy to report and control a growing array of communicable diseases.

Although Louisiana established the first state Board of Health in 1855, Massachusetts, in 1869, established what its historian describes as the "first in the United States to be based on a comprehensive program to prevent unnecessary mortality from all causes." General government in Massachusetts established the board in order to "reorganize and strengthen the administrative apparatus of government."[25] Establishing the board had initially been recommended in 1850, in a *Report of the Sanitary Condition of Massachusetts* by Lemuel Shattuck, a member and committee chair in the lower house of the legislature. In the ensuing decades, most of the other states created state and, usually, local health agencies.

States regulated medical licensure until the 1830s and 1840s, and then deregulated it. The competing theories of disease precluded consensus about appropriate medical interventions. Instead, a variety of what contemporaries called medical sects competed for patients. During the ascendance of Jacksonian Democracy in the 1830s and 1840s, advocates for these sects persuaded state officials that licensing laws unfairly protected elite physicians despite the absence of evidence of the effectiveness of their treatment.[26]

States reregulated licensing and professional discipline later in the century, mainly in response to organizations of physicians who associated themselves with recent advances in medical science, notably anesthesia and asepsis in surgery and the identification of bacterial causes of infectious disease. State medical societies, often joined by sectarian practitioners who competed with their members, lobbied to reestablish licensing boards and influenced appointments to them. Alabama even delegated regulatory authority to its state medical society; this delegation persists. States also established boards to regulate practitioners of other medical sects whose members continued to attract patients and contribute to election campaigns, notably osteopaths, chiropodists (subsequently called podiatrists), and chiropractors.[27]

Federal grants in aid accelerated states' centralization of what had previously been functions of local government and philanthropy. The first such program, under the Morrill Act of 1862, gave states federally owned land and authorized them to sell it to finance public colleges and universities. The scope and size of grant programs increased substantially during the Progressive Era and grew even more rapidly during the New Deal and after World War II. Between 1878 and 1921, Congress established six grant programs to address disease control, the safety of food and drugs, and maternal and child health. By the 1950s, grants assisted states in centralizing public health work, the planning and construction of hospitals, and the provision of health and social services to the indigent.[28]

Scholars disagree about the history of grant programs. Derthick writes that grants have "prodded and helped the states in a modern civilizing mission" directed by the federal government, and especially by the executive branch. Grants, she claims, induced otherwise reluctant states to match funds, to "secure statewide uniformity in program operations, and to create "merit systems of personnel administration."[29] Johnson, in contrast, documents extensive collaboration between state officials and members of Congress in designing and enacting grant programs and the broad discretionary authority that states retained.[30]

Federal grants were not, however, the sole or even the major cause of increased activism by state government in health affairs in the first four decades of the twentieth century. States made health policy mainly in response to the incidence and prevalence and, perhaps more important, risk of illness and injury in a growing population that often did dangerous work, ingested adulterated food and drugs, and had inadequate housing and sanitation.

By the 1890s, new scientific evidence was informing health policy in the states and major cities. This evidence demonstrated, for example, the effectiveness of vaccination against rabies, the success of an anti-toxin to treat diphtheria, and the reduced transmission of tuberculosis within households as a result of interventions by nurses and social workers. State agencies collaborated with local officials and civic leaders, and sometimes with charitable organizations as well, to make and implement health policy. Contrary to Derthick's claim, state health departments frequently sought uniformity in programs conducted by city and county government before federal grants became available for this purpose. Similarly, Progressives in many states did not need encouragement from the federal government to lobby for merit appointments, especially for professionals in departments of health.

Contrary to Progressive ideology, however, political patronage did not invariably cause the appointment of unqualified officials. For example, Tammany Hall, the Democratic Party machine in New York City and State gave sustained support to Hermann N. Biggs, an internationally renowned pathologist, researcher, and innovator in public health. After leading the health department in New York City for many years, Biggs, reorganized the State Department of Health in the second decade of the twentieth century.[31]

Tammany approved of officials whose scientific knowledge could improve the health of its voters and their families. In the mid-1890s, research, policy, and machine politics had converged in New York City. Biggs wanted to identify persons who had active tuberculosis in order to reduce their opportunities to infect others, especially in crowded tenement homes. He persuaded the city's Board of Health to require physicians to report cases of suspected tuberculosis and to initiate a program in a new city laboratory to test sputum for the bacterium that caused the disease. Biggs also established a program of home visiting of persons with confirmed cases of the disease. The Health Department employed interpreters who spoke more than thirty languages to accompany its professionals on these visits.

The New York County Medical Society protested these intrusions into its members' clinical practice. It particularly denounced the requirement to report cases of the disease and lobbied the state legislature to limit the authority of the city's Health Department.

Tammany defused the protest. At Biggs's suggestion, it facilitated an appropriation by the city's legislative body to the Health Department for a new program to inspect schoolchildren for evidence of disease. Under this program, more than one hundred members of the county medical society received stipends for part-time jobs inspecting children. This cash was particularly welcome because more physicians were practicing in the city than patients' fees could support during a severe national economic depression. The machine also intervened to prevent the state legislature from passing a bill to prohibit mandatory reporting of disease.

Scholars who assume that the federal government led reluctant and even incompetent states also ignore evidence that state and local government spent considerably more than the federal government did for health during the first two-thirds of the twentieth century. States welcomed federal grants because they supported their own goals. The Sheppard Towner Act for maternal and child health, enacted in 1921 and repealed in 1929 as a result of opposition from organized medicine, augmented many existing programs financed by states and public charities; thirty-four states had child health programs before 1920.[32] The Social Security Act of 1935 provided grants to expand and restore spending for existing state public health programs, especially in the 80 percent of counties that lacked full-time health staff.[33] The Hill-Burton Act of 1946 provided grants to construct and equip hospitals and to encourage regionalization of health services. States had been inspecting and subsidizing hospitals since the nineteenth century and encouraging the regional aspirations of the medical schools and teaching hospitals of public universities since the 1920s.[34]

Data about spending by states illustrate the extent to which their policy was independent of federal grants. During the 1920s, for instance, state revenues accounted for 80 percent of spending under federal grant programs. In 1938, despite diminished revenue as a result of the Depression, states accounted for 81 percent of all public spending for health care and hospitals. By comparison, state spending for welfare programs (mostly poor relief) was 87 percent of the total. Educational costs were 94 percent of the total.[35]

States' aggregate spending continued to exceed their revenue from federal funds. In 1955, for instance, federal grants in aid were only 31.7 percent of the total expenditures of state and local government. In 1988, after a quarter century of the most systematic nationalization of government functions in American history, federal grants to states had fallen to 18.2 percent of total spending.

Federal spending for health services began to exceed state expenditures after the implementation of Medicare and Medicaid. In 1960, states accounted for 14.3 percent of total health expenditures compared to only 10.4 percent for the federal government. In 1966, when Medicare and Medicaid were implemented, state spending fell 3 percent below federal for the first time; by 2006 federal spending for health services exceeded that of the states by 21 percent.[36]

States' spending for health services remained significant. Between 1960 and 2006 national health spending increased from just under $50 billion to just over $2 trillion; from 5.2 percent to 16 percent of Gross Domestic Product. The percentage spent by the states in each of these years was between 12.6 percent and 14.3 percent of the total. Cash expenditures demonstrate the influence of states' spending on health affairs. States spent $3.9 billion for health in 1960; and $265 billion in 2006. Adjusting for inflation, states spent almost 30 percent more in 2006 than in 1960.

THE EXPANSION OF STATE HEALTH POLICY AFTER WORLD WAR II

During the 1940s and 1950s, government in the states met surging demand for higher education for the health professions. The rapid growth of private health insurance was creating well-paid jobs in the health sector. Many returning veterans wanted careers as health professionals. Moreover, many general practitioners wanted to train in a specialty in order to attain higher incomes and better working conditions. Federal benefits for veterans under the G.I. Bill of Rights subsidized some of the demand for higher education for the health professions. But states used their own revenues to meet most of it.

States were the principal funders of all higher education. Between the 1940s and the 1980s, public and private expenditures for postsecondary education increased nearly ten times (adjusted for inflation). Over this generation, public appropriations for higher education increased from less than half to two-thirds of total spending. The federal share of spending for public higher education doubled in this period; the states' share tripled.[37]

State subsidies to educate health professionals grew rapidly. Many states created new or enlarged schools in public universities. Many also subsidized capital financing for new facilities for professional education and patient care in private universities.

State policy to enlarge the health workforce drew policymakers into related issues of health policy. By the end of the 1950s, state officials were seeking ways to increase the supply of physicians and dentists in under-served rural and inner-city areas. In the 1960s, they sought to address growing problems of access to primary care as a result of the preference of most medical school graduates to practice specialties.

State appropriations to educate nurses and allied health professionals subsidized, indirectly, more health services and increased their cost. These programs replaced hospital-based training that combined apprenticeship with technical education and usually led to certification rather than to degrees.

Although academic programs in nursing and the allied health profes-sions deprived hospitals of inexpensive labor, physicians and managers found it in their interest to support them. State appropriations for higher education saved hospitals the expense of classroom and laboratory educa-tion, which insurance plans were reluctant to reimburse.

Physicians and hospital managers also had incentives to support enroll-ment growth in these new academic programs. The number of allied professions was increasing as a result of advances in technology. These new practitioners made it possible for physicians to order more reimburs-able procedures. A growing supply of nurses reduced pressure on hospitals to increase their wages.

Beginning in the 1950s, education for the health professions expanded more rapidly than general higher education. Spending for medical educa-tion alone, adjusted for inflation, increased more than thirty times in the first four decades after World War II. States spent most of this money. Forty new allopathic medical schools, most of them in state university systems, opened after 1960, compared with sixteen in the previous half century. The number of osteopathic schools also increased as the education and work of allopaths and osteopaths became similar; one university (Michigan State) established allopathic and osteopathic schools on the same campus. Programs in allied health and nursing in colleges and uni-versities increased fivefold between the 1950s and the 1980s. By the early 1980s, state appropriations for each student preparing for a health profes-sion were, on average, five times greater than for students in other pro-grams in research universities, and more than ten times those for students in other programs of colleges that only awarded bachelor degrees.

Federal subsidies to educate health professionals augmented state appro-priations after Congress passed the Health Professions Education Assistance Act (HPEA) in 1963. Unlike federal grant programs that stimulated state spending, HPEA funds frequently supplemented it—for instance, to construct educational facilities and subsidize education in primary care. After the enactment of Medicare, federal payments to teaching hospitals for the salaries and supervision of interns, residents, and clinical fellows exceeded but did not replace state spending for this segment of the workforce. Moreover, state subsidies always exceeded federal grant funds for undergraduate medical and dental education, as well as for education in nursing and the allied health professions. The education of physicians' assistants (PAs) in the early 1970s was, briefly, an exception. New programs to educate PAs began with substantial federal funding as a result of both the shortage of primary care practitioners and of policy to assist combat medics returning from Vietnam to work in the civilian health sector.

The interns, residents and fellows who were paid with Medicare funds trained in hospitals and clinics that received substantial funding from states. Between the 1960s and the 1980s, for example, states provided almost two-thirds of the capital for facilities in which students in the health professions received clinical instruction. The federal-state Medicaid program was the source of a larger percentage of the revenue of teaching hospitals than of most community hospitals.

The academic health centers (AHCs) discussed in the previous chapter because of their influence on health services research exemplified the interrelatedness of different aspects of state health policy. States wanted AHCs to make hospitals and physicians in their regions more efficient and effective; to educate health professionals, most of whom would subsequently supply the regional workforce; and to conduct biomedical research, some of which could be commercialized.

AHCs made significant contributions to state and regional economies. In 1940, each dollar of economic activity generated by a public medical school, its hospitals, and its clinics cost a state about 35 cents in appropriations. By 1994, states spent about 15 cents for each dollar of regional economic activity generated by medical schools and academic health centers. Since then the return on state spending has increased, because state support of AHCS has declined while their budgets have continued to grow.

MAKING AND IMPLEMENTING HEALTH POLICY IN STATE GOVERNMENT, 1970–1990

The activity and authority of state government in health affairs changed substantially after the late 1960s because the enactment of Medicaid coincided with the transfer of electoral power to suburban voters and the

changes in legislatures described in Chapter 1. Suburbanites, now a substantial majority of Americans, demanded more and more effective public
services, including health services that applied advances in research to
increasingly prevalent chronic diseases. Legislative reapportionment in
response to decisions by the US Supreme court in *Baker v. Carr* (1962) and
Reynolds v. Sims (1964) empowered suburban voters.[38] Reapportionment
also brought into general government people from a greater variety of
occupations, as well as more women and members of minority groups.

Although governors and legislatures had been making health policy
since the nineteenth century, for most of that time few state employees
were experts on health. During the first half of the twentieth century the
only state employees who had expertise in health affairs were public health
physicians, engineers responsible for water quality, epidemiologists, and
the physicians and nurses who worked in state hospitals for persons with
mental illness, tuberculosis, and developmental disabilities. Generalists in
government usually deferred to these specialists.

Many of the experts on public health appointed by officials of general
government in cities, counties, and states expected those to whom they
were accountable to defer to their expertise and dedication to the public
good. For many years, specialists in public health have been taught in
graduate school and entry-level jobs that health policy is different from
other policy domains because it has a scientific basis and addresses disease,
suffering, life and death. Beginning with the rapid increase in the effectiveness of general government through what the pioneering scholar of public
administration Leonard White called "newly devised systems of centralized [financial] control" in the second and third decades of the century,
many specialists in public health have complained that generalists lacked
"specialized knowledge" and hence "sympathetic understanding."[39]
General government should, therefore, exempt public health officials from
the rules of normal politics. For example, a former New York City health
commissioner, contrasting her experience under Mayor John Lindsay in
the 1960s with that of her predecessor during the 1950s, said that "Mayor
Wagner gave Leona [Baumgartner] everything she asked for and she never
had to play politics." There is, however, much documentary evidence of
Baumgartner's political skill.

A substantial number of public health officials continued to expect
special treatment long after general government became the dominant
force in health policy. In the late 1990s, for instance, the chief executive
of a national association of public health officials, who had served in senior
positions in state and federal health agencies, proposed to erect highway

billboards advocating for more state funds for public health infrastructure. He was distressed to be advised that governors and legislators do not like to be lobbied on behalf of state employees. A decade later, a public health official insisted that science should inform policy. He demurred when advised to prepare a table displaying the relative strength of the evidence for each of the policies he endorsed to prevent a particular condition. The problem, he said, was that the evidence for some of the policies was weak or inconclusive.

Similarly, city, county, and state officials conducted a coordinated e-mail protest in 2001 against a report on health expenditures in the states by the National Association of Budget Officers (NASBO), whose members report to governors, and the Reforming States Group (RSG), whose members serve in general government.[40] Responsibility for such a report, seventy-five public health officials wrote, belonged in their agencies. Their form message received a form reply: that many people have opinions about what states have spent, but that the opinions that count are those of budget directors.

Generalists in state government frequently defer to public health officials because they respect their science-based expertise. In contrast, when they defer to leaders of the medical profession, they do so as a matter of politics. Many elected officials have had painful experience of physicians' defense of their autonomy. In the congressional elections of 1950, for example, the AMA and state medical societies took credit for defeating several incumbents, including the Senate majority leader, who supported national health insurance.[41] State medical societies have frequently criticized many legislators active in health policy as ignorant and interfering, accusing them of practicing medicine without a license.

But physicians' power has, increasingly, been limited. Many legislators and governors have offered persuasive incentives to leaders of organized medicine to remain neutral about particular policies or to negotiate rather than protest. The most important of these incentives was cooperation with the profession in protecting its clinical autonomy and especially the division of authority between community and academic physicians. Governors, for instance, consulted leaders of state and county medical societies about prospective appointees to the state boards that licensed and disciplined their colleagues.

Legislators who chaired health committees earned political credit with physicians by their reluctance to amend statutes that regulated the practice of health professionals. For example, they frequently delayed or avoided holding hearings on amendments to these laws sought by members of professions that wanted to expand the scope of their practice at physicians' expense; optometrists, nurse practitioners, and physical therapists, for example. Physicians avoided competition; legislators avoided protracted conflict.

The governing board of a state medical society provided an example of physicians' willingness to cooperate with state government in the mid-1980s. A state official described to the board a new center to assess health technology organized by the Department of Health in collaboration with the state university. The official said disingenuously that the technology assessments produced by the center were unlikely to influence Medicaid policy for covering technology.[42] The trustees agreed to remain neutral unless they received a large number of complaints that Medicaid officials were using the center's reports to deny coverage for drugs or devices that their members prescribed.

Another agenda item at this meeting demonstrated that physicians' lack of political discipline could impede the effectiveness of their advocacy. A representative of the lobbying firm retained by the society complained that many of the physician volunteers who assisted the firm made derogatory remarks to legislators about trial lawyers. He asked the trustees to inform the volunteers that trial lawyers were major contributors to the majority party in the lower chamber and that several of them were in the leadership of both chambers. The trustees said that they found it difficult to control the behavior of their members.

Since the 1960s, however, significant aspects of health policy have become too important to too many voters to be decided mainly in negotiations between state officials and representatives of health sector interest groups. Decisions about health policy transcended interest group politics for two reasons: they had important consequence for jobs, income, educational opportunity, and access to care, and rising expenditures for health services impeded spending for other public purposes. Sometimes states could pass laws that served the broad public interest when the federal government could not. For example, by 1984, every state had enacted a law permitting physicians and pharmacists to substitute generic for brand-name drugs; the pharmaceutical lobby continued to prevent passage of a substitution law by Congress.[43]

States' decisions about whether and where to build and how rapidly to expand AHCs exemplified the broad political importance of health policy. The construction industry and craft unions wanted lucrative contracts and subcontracts to build facilities for patient care, research, and teaching. Investors in real estate and their allies in the retail and home-building industries expected AHCs to stimulate new housing, shops, hotels, and technology parks. Local officials anticipated the property taxes paid by the highly paid health professionals and managers recruited to AHCs from other states and regions. Many voters aspired to lucrative and recession-proof jobs in health organizations. Parents and their adolescent children wanted more educational opportunities. Everyone hoped to experience state-of-the-art care for serious illness and injuries.

The interest groups and voters supporting the expansion of AHCs were more important to generalists in government than organizations of physicians and hospitals. During the 1960s and 1970s, these policymakers heard many complaints about the growth of AHCs from executives and trustees of community hospitals and many of the physicians who practiced in them. They told legislators and governors that they feared losing patients and hence income to academic physicians and teaching hospitals. State medical societies frequently and dental societies always feared that graduates of new or expanding schools would compete with their members.

After listening to such complaints, legislators and governors usually flashed a campaign smile and thanked their visitors for their comments. But they regularly asked officials of academic centers what they were doing to mollify their health sector colleagues. Mollifying tactics included raising the prestige of local physicians by offering them voluntary faculty appointments, adding rotations in community hospitals to university-based residency training programs, and negotiating vague agreements about the referral of patients from community hospitals and members of their medical staff. By the 1980s, most state university AHCs had a clinical faculty of between 250 and 400 full-time equivalent physicians in clinical disciplines and a voluntary faculty of 1,200 to 2,000 community physicians. Divided authority in the medical profession was becoming blurred authority in a political context in which state government was increasingly powerful.

Government generalists' knowledge about technical issues in policy for health care and professional education rapidly increased. Governors' budget staff sought comparative data about the number of faculty required to teach and provide clinical services in each profession and clinical discipline and the compensation of faculty at each rank in clinical and basic science disciplines. Budget and legislative staff demanded that AHCs provide evidence about projected demand for new services, beds, and students. They used their control over appropriations to punish AHC managers whom they caught offering self-serving information. Budget officials in one state learned, for instance, that two of its four public medical schools reported different data about the number of full-time equivalent faculty members to the Association of American Medical Colleges (AAMC) and the central administration of the state's university: higher numbers to AAMC to seek prestige; lower to the central administration to justify a larger appropriation.

Institutional characteristics of government in many states had made it difficult for legislators to increase their expertise in health policy during the 1950s and 1960s. Most legislators were part-time "citizen legislators." In many states, individual legislators had no staff, committee staffs were small, and the fiscal and research offices that served a chamber or the entire legislature were fully occupied with questions about revenue and expenditures in other areas than health. Many legislatures met every two years.

Governors also struggled with structural problems as health spending escalated. In some states, commissions, whose members served staggered terms, rather than governors, appointed agency heads. In others, legislatures limited the size of governors' direct staff. In one industrial state, requests for out-of-state travel required approval from the Governor's Council, which met only on Thursdays. If a federal official called on Friday to request a meeting in Washington the next Tuesday, a state employee risked an unreimbursed trip.

Despite these impediments, legislators and governors' staff quickly acquired expertise about Medicaid. Medicaid was legally complex because federal law and regulations combined modern concepts of insurance coverage for health services with statutory and case law that had accumulated since the early seventeenth century, when Britain enacted the Elizabethan Poor Law and extended it to its colonies.[44] Medicaid was also fiscally complex. The formula that established the percentage of each state's spending matched by the federal government took into account both economic conditions and the incidence of poverty. Ambiguities in the federal definition of allowable state expenditures for Medicaid became incentives to state officials to interpret accounting conventions creatively in order to maximize reimbursement.

Under Medicaid, moreover, states had considerable discretion about whom and what services to cover and how much to pay providers.[45] States set income thresholds for covering children and adults. They also defined medical indigence by setting the level of income and assets below which frail seniors and persons of all ages who had disabling conditions became eligible for Medicaid. Federal law mandated a minimum set of services, but states could cover additional services and receive matching funds for them. Moreover, states could propose waivers of federal regulations that permitted them to reorganize services if they could demonstrate budget neutrality. Some of these waiver programs eventually became national Medicaid policy, notably in managing AIDs/HIV and other diseases and for long-term care for frail seniors. States also set fees for the services of physicians and other health professionals, decided which pharmaceutical drugs and assistive devices to cover, and established reimbursement rates for hospital and nursing home stays and home visits by nurses and aides.

Medicare and Medicaid made what had been charity care lucrative. As a result, physicians and hospitals pressed states to subsidize the proliferation of services. By the early 1970s, almost any hospital that could recruit and equip specialists in surgery, cardiology, and gastro-intestinal medicine could obtain approval to open new services from state and regional planning agencies and equip them by selling tax-exempt bonds issued by public authorities created by legislatures.

By the end of the 1970s, the hierarchies of providers led by AHCs that had begun to emerge in the 1950s and 1960s existed mainly in universities' master plans and promotional brochures. Health planners and authors of textbooks on health administration had since the 1920s diagrammed these regional hierarchies as pyramids, with teaching hospitals and medical schools at their apex.[46] Half a century later, optimists diagrammed interinstitutional relationships as networks; pessimists complained about fragmentation.

Chapter 2 described the consequences of the failure to implement the theory of hierarchical regionalism for research on health services. Now I describe how this failure affected health policy more broadly.

The growing supply of reimbursable services in the absence of effective controls on which patients received what treatments in which settings accelerated cost inflation. By the mid-1970s, AHCs and community hospitals competed to perform many of the same procedures and the total number of lucrative services steadily increased.

Medicaid policy required constant attention from governors and legislators. The program affected the interests of most health professionals and institutional providers. Policy for Medicaid eligibility had become a priority for advocates on behalf of seniors, residents of low-income communities, and persons with disabilities.

THE POLITICS OF FEDERALISM, 1960–2000

The federal government complicated policymaking for health in the states by unprecedented efforts to centralize authority. Martha Derthick summarizes the history of centralization since the 1960s: "national programs, institutions, and techniques of influence came together to enlarge national power at state and local governments' expense [and as a result] federalism as a constitutional principle was sharply devalued." As examples, she cited the "critically important domains of civil rights, schools, police, and legislative districting."[47] A report by the Advisory Commission on Intergovernmental Relations in the mid-1980s concluded that "federal policymakers [have] turned increasingly to new, more intrusive and more compulsory regulatory programs to work their will."[48]

Federal intrusion was an additional incentive for state officials to increase their competence in making and implementing policy. In response to federal centralization, leaders of general government accelerated the structural reforms in the executive and legislative branches that had begun in the 1940s and 1950s. They also increased the number of highly skilled officials employed by agencies of specialized government.[49]

In the first four decades after World War II, the number of state employees tripled. Each state reorganized its executive branch. Twenty-eight states had replaced agencies headed by boards, commissions and elected officials with a cabinet in which agency heads reported to the governor by 1965. Over the next quarter century, twenty-six states undertook comprehensive administrative reorganization. Some states chartered public benefit corporations to manage state university teaching hospitals and clinics more effectively. Every state reorganized its procurement processes and human resources management and strengthened oversight of spending by state agencies and local government. To accomplish all this every state diversified its sources of revenue.

Legislative reform was also profound. Thirty-six legislatures held annual sessions by 1971; the number increased to forty-three by the 1990s. The percentage of legislators who were women and members of minority groups increased substantially. The percentage of attorneys fell; that of teachers and businesspeople increased.

Legislatures became so prominent in policymaking by the 1990s that conservative reformers campaigned for term limits in the states that had, since the Progressive Era, permitted citizens to initiate laws by petition and make them by referendum. Term-limit ballot measures succeeded in twenty-two states, mainly because of support for them from disgruntled citizens, many of whom thought they were voting to limit the terms of members of Congress rather than state legislators, but some of it from business groups that preferred to lobby less experienced legislators. Several states subsequently reversed term limits; only fifteen states still had them by 2007.[50]

No reforms could protect states from the effects of federal laws that preempted their authority to make policy. Congress has enacted statutes preempting state action since 1789, more than three-quarters of them since 1930. Between 1965 and 2004, it enacted 355 such statutes.[51]

Legal experts identify many varieties of preemption. Some federal preemption, for example, permits state law to supersede federal law if the state sets standards that equal or exceed national standards; other preemption statutes combine federal and state regulation, or allow the federal government to transfer regulatory authority to states that have laws consistent with federal standards. Preemption can also be implicit in federal law—for example, where federal law and regulation is "so pervasive as to make reasonable the inference that Congress left no room for the states to supplement it," or when "compliance with both federal and state regulations is a physical impossibility" or "a state law impedes the accomplishment of a federal goal or objective."[52]

The politics of preemption is mainly about money. Interest groups lobby Congress to preempt state laws in order to avoid the cost of regulation and litigation, or at least to centralize these costs.

Federal courts have usually sustained and strengthened preemptive legislation. A scholar of federal jurisprudence, assessing the history of preemption cases decided by the Supreme Court, concluded that these decisions reduced the sovereignty of states by making federalism a "political structure in which states' interests are . . . [merely] represented in the national political process."[53]

Complicated preemption language in the Employee Retirement Income Security Act of 1974 (ERISA) has severely limited states' ability to expand access to health care. ERISA preempted state authority to regulate employee benefit plans. But states retained authority to regulate the "business of insurance." Therefore, employers that financed employee benefit plans as defined in ERISA could, by self-insuring, become exempt from state regulation. The interest groups that supported ERISA preemption also succeeded for over two decades in preventing any federal regulation of the health coverage offered by employee benefit plans. These plans enjoyed a regulatory vacuum in which they were free from intrusion by either the federal government or the states.

ERISA preemption of state regulation of self-insured coverage was controversial by the late 1970s. When ERISA became law in 1974, many policymakers and lobbyists had expected that the federal government would soon regulate health benefits in a parallel statute or enact national health insurance. But political stalemate prevented universal coverage. Large employers and unions that operated self-insured health plans because their members had multiple employers then became aggressive in protecting ERISA preemption. They effectively lobbied members of Congress to defeat proposals to regulate employee health plans or to grant exemptions from ERISA to enable individual states to regulate them. Hawaii won an exemption. But the conference committee that granted it explained in the formal legislative history that Hawaii's exemption would not be a precedent. Supporters of ERISA preemption also won many lawsuits against states that tried to circumvent it by artfully crafting statutes to expand access to health care.[54]

As a result of the politics of ERISA preemption, neither the federal government nor the states regulate the coverage offered by the health plans in which most insured employees are enrolled. A study in 1996 found that 40 percent of all covered employees, and 60 percent in the largest firms, were in self-insured plans. By 2000, 49 percent of covered employees were in such plans. By 2007, the number had risen to 55 percent.[55]

THE STATES AND HEALTH REFORM SINCE 1990

ERISA preemption frustrated the governors and legislative leaders who had, in the late 1980s, mobilized support for policy to expand access to health care by giving employers a choice of either covering their employees or paying a tax that states would use to purchase coverage for them. The failure of the Clinton health reform plan in 1993–94, which would have superseded ERISA preemption, added to their frustration.

Nevertheless, leaders in many states continued to enact significant advances in health policy and to press for changes in federal law. In the late 1980s and early 1990s, seven states enacted statutes to increase access to care: Florida, Maryland, Massachusetts, Minnesota, Oregon, Vermont, and Washington. Hawaii had expanded access earlier under its waiver of ERISA preemption. In many of these states executives of some large firms that self-insured supported access reform. They reasoned that reducing the number of uninsured persons would reduce the cost to employers of cross-subsidizing uncompensated hospital care. This support did not, however, offset opposition to Congress granting exemptions from ERISA from corporations and craft unions joined by associations representing small business.[56]

The "reforming states," a name they took in 1993, expanded access to care to the limit permitted by ERISA preemption.[57] Minnesota, for example, taxed the revenues of hospitals and physicians to pay for more coverage for low-income families because it could not tax employers' health plans. Maryland devised and marketed through a state commission affordable minimum coverage by commercial health insurance policies for persons employed in small business and their dependents. Vermont covered more children with more services paid by Medicaid and state appropriations. Oregon expanded enrolment in Medicaid at an affordable cost by rationing coverage through a public deliberative process and also subsidized insurance for the working poor.

In 1993 and 1994, leaders of general government from the reforming states invited colleagues from other states to join them to discuss what they were learning from policy to expand access and how to concert their efforts to influence federal policy. Calling themselves the Reforming States Group (RSG), they arranged meetings with members of Congress and White House staff to discuss how federal policy could help states expand access to care. Following a lunch meeting of RSG legislators with the Senate Democratic Caucus in May 1994, Senator Tom Daschle (D-S.D.), then chairman of the Democratic Policy Committee, wrote his colleagues that the visitors "made some points that are very important to the effort in which we are now involved." He emphasized the importance of evidence presented by the RSG that a growing number of national and multinational corporations would support mandatory health insurance.[58] Daschle told a member of the RSG that his colleagues had stayed longer and been unusually attentive because these state legislators had "enacted health reform and been re-elected."

During the spring and summer of 1994, RSG members, now from fourteen states, negotiated an alternative to the rapidly failing Clinton health plan with members of Congress, their staff, and representatives of thirty Fortune 100 employers. Under this plan self-insured employers would remain exempt from state regulation and from taxes on insurance premiums to protect against catastrophic risks. In return, these employers would endorse a new federal tax on business, the revenue from which would be distributed to states that enacted universal coverage. This compromise was included in an alternative health reform bill submitted in August by Senate Majority Leader George Mitchell (D-Maine) and Senator John Chafee (R-R.I.) and reported in the national press.[59] Mitchell withdrew the bill in September, however, because the White House would not support it, even after the defeat of its own plan, and because many

Republicans were reluctant to give Democrats a victory on health reform two months before Election Day.

Leaders of general government in many states continued to press for health reform. During the next several years, many states broadened eligibility and coverage in their Medicaid programs and increased subsidies to insure children and to help seniors with low incomes pay for prescription drugs.

State officials also continued to work with large corporations. Medicaid recipients, public employees, and employees of large firms comprised at least half the population with health coverage in most states. Government and employers could potentially use their substantial countervailing power to press health plans and provider organizations to contain costs and improve the quality of care. But many employers hesitated to join states in asserting such countervailing power; some because of ideological discomfort with government, others because they believed that the third-party administrators of their self-insured plans were negotiating the lowest possible physicians' fees, hospital rates and prescription prices.

Many employers, however, encouraged greater oversight by state government of the solvency and honesty of organizations in the health sector and the quality of the care they provided; especially managed care plans. Although these plans contained costs, consumer backlash against their delays and denials of coverage caused many labor unions and individual employees to complain to corporate executives. Acting on justified complaints could cause the rate of increase in the cost of health benefits to once again rise above the rate of inflation in the general economy. A 1996 study of state oversight of integrated health systems by the RSG documented that many states had taken advantage of business support to increase the accountability of health plans and providers.[60]

Members of the RSG and the national associations of governors and legislators continued to advocate on behalf of expanded access to care to Congress and the federal executive branch. RSG members testified, for example, in favor of what became the Health Insurance Portability and Accountability Act of 1996 (HIPAA). This was the first legislation to puncture the regulatory vacuum created by ERISA preemption. RSG members also supported the first federal legislation to require partial parity between coverage for mental illness and other conditions, which also eroded ERISA preemption. They regularly discussed changes in regulations with senior federal officials responsible for Medicaid.

In 1997, the RSG responded to a request for assistance in drafting legislation to create the State Children's Health Insurance Program (SCHIP) from Paul Harrington, staff director of the Senate Committee on Health, Education, Labor and Pensions. Harrington had participated in the RSG as a legislator in Vermont and then as one of three members of the commission that implemented the state's legislation to expand access. He had been one of the RSG members who met with members of Congress to discuss health reform in 1993 and 1994.

Harrington asked the RSG, on behalf of James Jeffords (R-Vt.), the chair of the Senate Committee, for help in resolving a dispute about the scope of benefits that threatened to prevent the passage of SCHIP. The National Governors Association wanted states to determine benefits. Organizations that advocated on behalf of children wanted SCHIP to provide each enrollee with enhanced and expensive Medicaid coverage that was currently available to the poorest children under a program called Early Periodic Screening, Detection and Treatment (EPSDT).

RSG members from ten states devised four benefit plans and recommended that SCHIP permit each state to choose one of them. The plans ranged in scope from EPSDT to the coverage currently available to dependents of a state's public employees. The RSG members described and justified these alternative benefits in a letter to the House and Senate co-chairs of the conference committee that was negotiating the details of SCHIP. Harrington participated in the meeting at which the conferees discussed and accepted the RSG's recommendation. He said subsequently that the letter had been "definitive" in the passage of SCHIP. The conferees, he added, appreciated the recommended compromise and took particular notice of the names and official positions of the members of the RSG Steering Committee. By 2007, SCHIP covered six million children.

THE RELEVANCE OF RESEARCH TO STATES IN THE RECESSION OF 2001

Most members of the RSG remained eager to expand access to health care. They were also committed to protecting the access that had been achieved. The recession of 2000–2001 threatened to diminish access because it reduced states' revenues.

Recessions have more severe consequences for states than for the federal government because the constitutions of forty-nine of them require balanced budgets. States have broadened the definition of balance to include borrowed funds, one-time payments, lagged payrolls and employee furloughs. But declining tax revenues invariably require them to spend less.

Health was the largest object of expenditure by the states in fiscal years 2000 and 2001. Programs of direct services combined with spending for population health accounted for 30 percent of state budgets; Medicaid alone was 19.6 percent. In the same fiscal years the next largest expenditures were for elementary and secondary education, 22.2 percent, and higher education, 11.3 percent. In 2001, thirty-seven states reduced their budgets by about 5 percent, a total of $13 billion.[61]

State spending for pharmaceutical drugs was increasing faster than for any other covered service. States paid for drugs for Medicaid and SCHIP beneficiaries, for persons receiving care under Workers' Compensation, and for current and retired state employees and their dependents. Thirty-four states subsidized the purchase of essential drugs by seniors with low incomes. By 2002, when states began to implement preferred drug lists (PDLs), they were spending $30 billion a year to purchase prescription drugs; almost a seventh of total state expenditures for health services.[62]

State officials ascribed escalating drug costs to factors that included, as the RSG Steering Committee wrote in *Health Affairs*, "an aging population, unit price increases for existing drug products, the introduction of new, more expensive agents, widespread marketing efforts by manufacturers, advocacy by various interests, and increases in the use of drugs as a substitute for other health services." The Steering Committee also criticized federal Medicaid regulations governing rebates to them from pharmaceutical manufacturers for obscuring the prices paid by each state. Moreover, it deplored policies of the Food and Drug Administration that inhibited "timely, accurate, and independent information for prescribers and purchasers on the relative effectiveness of different pharmaceutical agents."

The underlying cause of rising costs, the state officials said, was a "dysfunctional market in which information on price and relative effectiveness either is not available or is obscured."[63] They then described programs in five states to contain the increase in drug costs and several multi-state initiatives. Two of the states, Michigan and Oregon, had recently initiated PDLs that made decisions informed by independent research. A federal court had recently upheld the Michigan program against a challenge from the pharmaceutical industry. Science and politics were about to converge to yield more effective policy.

4. The Drug Effectiveness Review Project

Research on health services and policymaking converged in 2001 when states began to use systematic reviews to inform decisions about covering pharmaceutical drugs for Medicaid programs. Chapter 1 summarized the immediate and underlying causes of this convergence. Chapter 2 described how the politics of the health sector in the United States has influenced the questions and methods of health services research. Chapter 3 explained the growth of states' responsibilities in health affairs. Chapters 2 and 3 both explained how senior legislators and officials of the executive branch in many states learned how research could inform policy. This chapter describes how and with what effects state officials are applying to policy the methods and findings of research on the effectiveness and comparative effectiveness of pharmaceutical drugs.

Because of my personal involvement in encouraging this convergence I risk readers' suspicion that I exaggerate its extent and its significance and understate its limitations and fragility. I am, however, both skeptical about the sustainability of convergence and delighted that I can tell this story. The next chapter is about my skepticism; this one is about my delight. As the minutes of the Second Annual Participant Governance Meeting of the Drug Effectiveness Review Project (DERP) in April 2004 record:

> Dan Fox . . . noted that if in the year 2000 anyone would have said that [research on the] effectiveness of health services will actually drive policy, he would not have believed it. It has been his dream— never believing it would happen in his lifetime. He remembered that Archie Cochrane's 1972 book was the first call for head-to-head effectiveness comparisons. It has become clear in the last several years that science has reached the point of being useful to policymakers and policymakers have reached the point of being willing and courageous [enough] to use science. And here we are. Wow.[1]

This quotation also illustrates another theme of this book; that the convergence of research and health policymaking in American states has, like most historical events, been contingent on human behavior and unexpected events.

ESTABLISHING THE DRUG EFFECTIVENESS REVIEW PROJECT

The convergence of science and health policymaking in the states was only a wish in 2000 despite advances in research methods and the increasing analytical competence of state government. I reported in Chapter 1 that in December 2000, John Santa, an Oregon official, had inquired about the PDL in British Columbia (called the Reference Drug Program) at a meeting of about forty policymakers from western states. None of his colleagues knew about this policy.

I explained to the western policymakers that officials in British Columbia and in a growing number of jurisdictions outside North America had begun in the 1990s to compare the effectiveness of drugs within particular classes using evidence from independent research. They listed as preferred the drugs in each class that were most effective and that had the lowest prices among equally effective competitors. They added drugs that were chemically equivalent to the preferred drugs to the lists when manufacturers lowered their prices to the level of the preferred drugs. Policymakers created incentives for physicians to prescribe the preferred drugs, most often by requiring them to obtain prior approval from a public agency to prescribe drugs that were not on the list. That was the end of the discussion.[2]

Andrew Oxman, then chair of the Cochrane Collaboration's Steering Group, and I had commissioned a case study of the PDL in British Columbia a year earlier for a report that would be published in 2001 as *Informing Judgment: Case Studies of Health Policy and Research in Six Countries*. We had no difficulty finding examples of convergence in Australia, Britain, Canada, and Norway. Each of these cases described public policy for prescribing prescription drugs that had been informed by research. But we could not identify any American state or federal agency in which researchers and policymakers routinely collaborated to use evidence-based health research to inform health policy. In the absence of a case from government, physicians and a policymaker at Kaiser Permanente wrote the American chapter of the report.[3]

Because Santa's query had provoked little interest, I did not say that several weeks earlier leading pharmaceutical manufacturers had denounced the scientific basis of policy for drug coverage in Australia, Britain, Canada, and Norway. The policymakers and researchers who wrote the case studies Oxman and I commissioned had met in October 2000 to review one another's drafts and discuss common themes. The authors of the case studies suspected that the attacks had occurred because a co-author of one of them, an employee of a pharmaceutical company, had leaked the embargoed drafts.

The attacks were particularly effective in Australia and Britain. In Australia, industry pressure caused the government to reorganize the policy-making Australian Benefits Advisory Committee. David Henry, the co-author of one of the case studies, lost his position. The country's highest court subsequently reaffirmed the process by which the committee had been making policy and vindicated Henry. In Britain, the National Institute for Clinical Excellence (NICE) changed its recommendation against covering Relenza, a treatment for influenza that was the subject of the case study. In Norway, in contrast, angry senior civil servants denounced the attacks to the media and were supported by elected officials.

A substantial projected increase in Oregon's Medicaid budget for fiscal year 2001 had prompted Santa's question about the PDL in British Columbia. Prescription drugs were the fastest growing segment of that budget. Their cost had increased by 60 percent during the previous two years, Governor John Kitzhaber told the legislature. Oregon was typical. The cost of prescription drugs as a percentage of the total cost of Medicaid across the country more than doubled from 5.6 percent in 1992 to 12 percent in 2002.[4]

Oregon officials soon adapted lessons from British Columbia to local political conditions. In February 2001, Mark Gibson, the governor's policy adviser for health and social policy, invited Bob Nakagawa, the British Columbia official who had designed its PDL, to the capitol in Salem, as noted in Chapter 1. Then the governor's staff drafted a bill that would enable the executive branch to use peer-reviewed medical literature to inform policy for covering drugs for Medicaid and eventually for other state programs. To appeal to physicians' professionalism, they called the initiative the Practitioner-managed Prescription Drug Plan.

The legislation authorized an existing state advisory commission, most of the members of which were physicians, to interpret the evidence in each review and make recommendations to the state's Medicaid agency about the relative effectiveness of the drugs in each class. To prevent them from being influenced by any criteria except maximizing benefits to patients, commission members would not have access to data about the cost to the state of each drug. Moreover, unlike in British Columbia, the PDL would be advisory; physicians need not obtain prior authorization for nonpreferred drugs.

Members of the governor's staff were familiar with health services research. They had used it in ranking conditions and interventions in the Oregon Health Plan, which Governor Kitzhaber had initiated when he was Senate president. Moreover, several of them were acquainted with the methods and uses of systematic reviews. Mark Gibson (who subsequently would direct the DERP, in collaboration with Pam Curtis, John Santa, and then Allison Little), had participated in many meetings convened by both the User Liaison Program of the federal Agency for Health Care Research and Policy (AHCPR) and the Milbank Memorial Fund. He was also a founder of the Reforming States Group (RSG) and a participant in conversations among its members about the methods and uses of research. John Santa was a physician who had used the findings of international research on effectiveness as a staff member of the Technology Evaluation Center (TEC) of the Blue Cross and Blue Shield Association (BCBSA).

Santa introduced his colleagues on the governor's staff to Mark Helfand, a physician and researcher at the Oregon Health and Science University who conducted systematic reviews. Helfand directed one of the Evidence-based Practice Centers (EPCs) designated by AHCPR. The Oregon EPC had conducted systematic reviews for the U.S. Preventive Services Task Force and the Community Guide Program of the Centers for Disease Control and Prevention (CDC). Like his colleagues in other EPCs, Helfand followed the work of the Cochrane Collaboration. Similarly, Robert Brook, the director of another EPC that would work with DERP said in 2004, "We all use Cochrane as our starting point."[5]

The bill to create the Oregon PDL stalled in the legislature as a result of lobbying by pharmaceutical companies and patient advocacy groups to which the companies contributed funds. During the final week of the legislative session, in late July, Kitzhaber acted to encourage passage of the bill. According to Pam Curtis, then on his staff, the governor told legislative leaders that he was prepared to veto the state's entire human services budget and then conduct a public campaign on behalf of the bill, after which he would convene a special session of the legislature. The bill passed.

Policymakers from Idaho and Washington State soon began to collaborate with their Oregon colleagues to commission systematic reviews of drug classes. These states augmented funds appropriated in Oregon to conduct the reviews; all three states also used federal matching funds under Medicaid. The PDLs in Idaho and Washington required prior approval when physicians prescribed nonpreferred drugs.

By then other states were creating PDLs. Federal regulations governing Medicaid prohibited states from establishing formularies, lists of drugs that physicians could prescribe. But the regulations permitted them to designate particular drugs as preferred and to require prior authorization to prescribe unlisted drugs. The regulations also permitted states to invite manufacturers of drugs that were chemically equivalent to but more expensive than preferred drugs to acquire preferred status for their products by paying "supplemental rebates" to states; these rebates effectively reduced the cost of these drugs to that of the preferred drug.[6]

Most states, like many large group practices that established formularies, appointed committees of physicians and pharmacists to evaluate new drugs. These committees based their recommendations about coverage mainly on articles in medical journals evaluating individual drugs against placebos, on dossiers submitted by pharmaceutical companies that included evidence from clinical trials, reports of adverse events, and judgments about effectiveness, and on the informed opinions of the committees' members. In some states, companies called Pharmacy Benefit Managers (PBMs) supplemented this evidence. PBMs coordinated pharmaceutical purchasing for many Medicaid programs, as well as for health systems, insurers, and large self-insured companies. Most PBMs also received rebates from drug manufacturers, which they were not obligated to disclose to their customers.

The project that began in Oregon and expanded to become DERP conducted systematic reviews and made them available to these committees and to the policymakers they advised. A relatively small number of systematic reviews comparing drugs in classes had been published in the international literature since the 1970s. Their number had increased since the mid-1990s, to a large extent as a result of demand for them by policymakers in Australia, British Columbia, and the United Kingdom.

DERP added substantially to the supply of reviews of drug classes. It also made systematic reviews responsive to policymakers' priorities. Moreover, its methodology and commitment to external scientific review persuaded expert committees and policymakers to trust the independence and rigor of its findings.

Early in 2003, DERP's founders in Idaho, Oregon, and Washington invited colleagues from other jurisdictions to join them in a "self-governing collaboration" to conduct and disseminate systematic reviews of classes of drugs. They proposed that collaborating states finance the project for three years and prorate its cost. By November 2004 Alaska, Arkansas, Kansas, Michigan, Minnesota, Missouri, North Carolina, Wisconsin, and Wyoming had joined. Over the next few years, California, Montana, and New York joined. The California Healthcare Foundation (CHCF) joined on behalf of itself and the California Public Employees Retirement System (CalPERS). A Canadian intergovernmental agency (now called the Canadian Agency for Drugs and Technology in Health) joined on behalf of the federal government and the provinces. All but two of the states and CHCF subsequently renewed their membership for another three years. Colorado joined in 2008; Maryland in January 2009.

Because DERP made its systematic reviews publicly available without charge, they informed decisions in other states that created PDLs. AARP and Consumer's Union made DERP reviews available to the general public in accessible formats and free of charge.

A year after the inception of DERP a staff member of the National Conference of State Legislatures told the *New York Times* that twenty-six states had PDLs and "10 others have enacted legislation authorizing their use."[7] By 2008, thirty-three states had operating PDLs; nine were implementing them; in two others regulations to create PDLs "may be delayed or blocked."[8] Policy varied among the states. Some excluded classes from the PDLs (e.g., drugs for mental illness, hemophilia, and AIDS/HIV). Some states made prior approval easier to obtain then others. A few states required higher co-payments for nonpreferred drugs.

At the first annual "participant governance meeting" of DERP in October 2003, officials from fifteen jurisdictions agreed that their reasons for collaborating went beyond prioritizing and commissioning reviews to inform PDLs. These reasons included informing other regulatory processes, containing costs, sharing information among states, doing work that states could not do alone, informing legislators, and providing information to providers and consumers. Former Governor Kitzhaber told the group, "Today's problems are complicated and the solutions that are required involve[d] thousands of people whose behavior cannot be compelled with law or regulation."[9]

This generalization had particular significance for state officials participating in DERP. Each of them had direct experience of industry opposition to the creation of PDLs that would be informed by independent research. Each of them had also experienced or anticipated well-financed resistance to their states' joining DERP and using its reviews from the pharmaceutical industry, patient advocacy groups, and some organizations of physicians. Several states that had established PDLs decided against joining DERP in order to avoid further antagonizing the industry. After a presentation by Burness Communications, a nonprofit firm, on "communicating with external organizations," the collaborating states welcomed an offer from the Milbank Memorial Fund to contract with Burness to assist them. At the end of the meeting they requested "basic communications tools from Burness as soon as possible."[10]

HOW DERP DOES ITS WORK

"The governance," one representative of each participating jurisdiction or organization, makes policy for DERP in conference calls and face-to-face meetings. Staff at the Center for Evidence-based Policy at the Oregon Health and Science University implements this policy. The governance establishes the order in which classes of drugs are evaluated and existing reviews updated. Then its members solicit suggestions for key questions for each review from health professionals within their jurisdictions and work with researchers to select the questions and word them precisely. Staff commissions reviews and updates, posts questions and comments on them for public review, administers reviews by experts of drafts of reviews on drugs in a class, manages relationships with pharmaceutical companies and national advocacy groups, and posts completed reviews and updates of them on the Web for open access.

Policy evolved as the governance assessed its experience and responded to external suggestions and criticism. The most significant DERP policies addressed priority setting, conflicts of interest, defining key questions, the collection and evaluation of evidence, presenting findings from reviews, and relationships with the pharmaceutical industry and its surrogates.[11]

The list of criteria for setting priorities for reviewing classes of drugs grew over time. At their first meeting to select drug classes for review, in 2003, members' criteria for priority were the "percent of the pharmaceutical budget" a class absorbed, "classes with multiple drugs of similar action," evidence that drugs are "being used in an inappropriate fashion," the "political visibility" of a drug or class, drugs that attracted "a great deal of advocacy," the emergence of " 'me too' " drugs, and "evidence of very expensive drugs added to a class."[12]

By 2007, criteria for prioritizing reviews included more precise questions about the public interest in evaluating particular drug classes. Perhaps most important, the incidence and prevalence of the conditions treated with a class of drugs became a significant consideration for reviewing a class. The governance also considered whether a review could add value because of the availability of evidence about the comparative effectiveness of drugs and competing treatments.[13]

Members' increasing knowledge about the primary research evaluated in systematic reviews informed the priorities they established for updating them. At the beginning of DERP the governance scheduled updates of reviews at set intervals. By 2007, members were examining evidence about a drug or a class published in the previous three years before deciding whether an update would be helpful. In 2007, staff and members began to examine new primary studies of each drug class that had been reviewed annually for findings that could trigger updates.

DERP criteria for setting priorities for initial reviews and updates also took account of the intense interest of patients and their advocates, manufacturers, and physicians in which drugs public programs would prefer. The governance considered the budgetary impact of new and emerging drugs, the "aggressiveness of the marketing techniques" used by the industry, and policy or coverage issues that particular members might have. The latter included, for example, efforts by advocates and interest groups to exclude classes of drugs from PDLs and hence from evaluation.[14]

The governance adopted unusually rigorous standards for conflicts of interest at its first meeting. Most organizations that sponsor health research require investigators to disclose potential conflicts. But disclosure alone was an insufficient standard when the purpose of the research was to inform policy that affected millions of consumers and billions of dollars. Interest and advocacy groups were likely to use any conflicts disclosed by researchers or expert reviewers of a DERP report to discredit it. Therefore DERP required that "report authors and [the research and review] process . . . be 100 percent free of any potential conflict."[15]

The DERP governance also required its own members to "declare any potential, perceived or real conflict they may have to the group." A deputy secretary of a department of health and human services, for instance, declared a potential conflict at a DERP governance meeting in 2004. His state had "asked pharmaceutical companies to pay for part of the cost of [its] disease management program, approximately $6 million." The governance decided that the conflict was not "serious enough" to preclude his full participation in its deliberations.[16]

DERP also sought to deflect criticism by commissioning systematic reviews only from EPCs designated by the federal Agency for Healthcare Research and Quality (AHRQ; formerly AHCPR). Research organizations compete to become EPCs in order to be eligible to conduct reviews commissioned by AHRQ on behalf of collaborating federal agencies and external organizations. EPCs at RAND (for the first three years), the Research Triangle Institute, and the Oregon Health and Science University have produced reviews for DERP. The Oregon EPC coordinates their work.

DERP reports do not include recommendations about policy. A significant reason for avoiding recommendations is to preclude advocacy and interest groups from claiming that DERP's systematic reviews select evidence in order to support its recommendations.

DERP also declines to recommend policy because jurisdictions have different value preferences, politics, and resources. States and provinces make local decisions about which drugs to prefer on the basis of advice from formal committees and testimony from interested professionals and groups. The same evidence has, at times, supported different policies. For example, Gibson explained that "early on Oregon and Washington used the same review of triptans to reach different conclusions. Oregon decided to prefer Ritzatriptan, which relieved pain faster than Sumatriptan, another effective drug, because patients had told policymakers that their priority was relief from pain as soon as possible. Policymakers in Washington State chose both drugs for their list after "considering a broader array of clinical endpoints," Gibson said.[17] A Canadian policymaker made a similar point when she summarized how provinces use reports about effectiveness from that country's Common Drug Review: "No [ineffective] means no; yes [effective in particular circumstances] means maybe."[18]

Moreover, by limiting reports to findings from reviewing clinical evidence DERP's governance encouraged variety and creativity in how different jurisdictions and other organizations use them. In some states, DERP reports are the only information that committees consider in making decisions about preferred drugs. Other states use information provided by PBMs as well as by DERP and other sources. A few states use DERP reports for provider education, whether or not they have PDLs. The Canadian member distributes DERP reports to committees that advise on policy in the provinces and territories.

The governance decided that including economic evaluation in DERP reports would also limit their usefulness. States differ in how they use information about cost and cost-effectiveness in deciding which drugs to prefer. In some states a separate committee on cost makes final decisions about coverage; weighing information about savings from supplemental rebates against expert recommendations about comparative effectiveness.

In others, policymakers prioritize information about comparative effectiveness over data about cost.

Skepticism about combining economic evaluation with reviews of clinical evidence predates DERP. In one of the first articles by an American describing the potential influence of systematic reviews on policy, Fred Mosteller, a Harvard statistician, warned in 1993 that many "interests may not accept [cost-effectiveness analysis] as readily as a safety and efficacy program." Cost-effectiveness analysis should be conducted, he wrote, "but not under the same roof" as systematic reviews.[19] A decade later, a British economist reported that many policymakers preferred to "impute their own values to the costs and consequences of decisions" rather than accept studies based on values selected for them by external researchers.[20] In 2006, a committee of the Institute of Medicine of the National Academies of Science warned that quality-adjusted life years (QALYs), the method of measuring the cost-effectiveness of health services most frequently used, raise "an important and difficult set of distributive issues and choices."[21] One issue was that different methods of economic evaluation impute different values. QALYs value each year of life equally. But a competing metric designed by the World Bank, disability-adjusted life years (DALYS), values the lives of working-age adults more highly than those of infants or the elderly.[22]

Experts in cost-effectiveness analysis frequently take offense at such skepticism. An American economist, for instance, described DERP's policy as a symptom of broader national failure: "The DERP decision to ignore cost-effectiveness considerations reveals a society still unable to consider economic factors openly in evidence reviews."[23] A British economist who helped to develop QALYs was equally disdainful. In an e-mail message in 2005, he criticized Sir Iain Chalmers, founder of the Cochrane Collaboration, for not insisting that economic evaluation accompany each systematic review and "reprimand[ed]" the Milbank Fund [and me personally] for "furthering such myopia."[24]

DERP policy for acquiring and assessing evidence also demonstrated convergence of the methods of research and the politics of policymaking. Some participants in the Cochrane Collaboration have complained that the rapidly increasing number of systematic reviews in the world literature—2,500 a year by 2005—should enable DERP, on occasion, to rely on published reviews instead of commissioning its own. DERP takes account of published reviews that meet its inclusion criteria; but not, to date, as substitutes for reviews it could have commissioned from an EPC.

DERP relies mainly on reviews it commissions because there are few sources of systematic reviews that are relevant to coverage policy. The number of systematic reviews of drug classes has not increased rapidly enough to meet worldwide demand from policymakers. For example, the Australian Pharmacy Benefit Scheme (PBS), a pioneer in using independent evidence to inform coverage policy, was still relying mainly on less rigorous studies when American states began to establish PDLs. According to David Henry, systematic reviews, both published and conducted internally, informed only 28 percent of major coverage decisions in Australia by 1998, an increase from 18 percent five years earlier.[25] Ruth Lopert, an Australian physician and civil servant who is an experienced regulator of pharmaceutical drugs, said in 2008, "We don't use drug class reviews except on a few occasions; but we may infer a class relationship rather than do a formal review."[26]

In order to decide which drugs to prefer, officials in British Columbia had introduced critical appraisal, an essential aspect of systematic reviewing, in 1995. But they found relatively few systematic reviews that compared drugs with each other rather than with a placebo. Bob Nakagawa recalled that "in those days there was a large spread for prices for drugs within a class, so we needed to establish that we were prepared to pay for good outcomes not better marketing." He commissioned the British Columbia Therapeutic Initiative to "conduct our reviews [because] there was no other source . . . at the time."[27] Similarly, Andrew Oxman recalled that the motivation for an important early comparative review of a class of drugs was not a coverage decision but whether it is ethical to use placebo rather than active controls for a trial when there is "compelling evidence" that there is an effective intervention.[28]

Moreover, systematic reviews vary in their quality and hence their credibility. Researchers have, for example, established a relationship between the source of systematic reviews and their findings. Cochrane reviews are consistently less favorable to the interventions studied than commercially sponsored reviews, and even than reviews by other non-profit organizations. Moreover, the technical quality of reviews varies, especially their standards for including studies and the accuracy with which data are reported. Even reviews in the Cochrane Library vary in quality, though less widely than other published reviews.

When Mark Helfand began to conduct the first systematic reviews for the state of Oregon in 2001, he was familiar with both the unsystematic reviews most public and private organizations used in making coverage policy and with the international literature of systematic reviews. He was surprised at how few systematic reviews he found of drugs in particular classes. "Most reviews," he recalled, "covered one drug and one indication (e.g. 'eletriptan for migraine') rather than several." In conducting reviews that could inform policy, in contrast, "one starts with the presumption that a physician is considering using one of the drugs. The review addresses which one(s) are more effective and safer, not whether to use one at all."

Helfand described how DERP combined methodological rigor with responsiveness to policymakers. "What we did differently," he wrote in 2008, "was to create an entire library of reviews based on [several] principles." These principles were:

- . . . emphasize health outcomes rather than surrogates . . . [and then] identify claims underlying competition in the marketplace and translate these claims . . . into claims about clinical outcomes that can be tested

- Cover the range of indications and drugs [that] decision-makers will [consider] . . . in the context of preferred-drug or formulary decision making [and]

- Highlight head-to-head comparisons (and their absence)[29]

DERP also set different expectations for the productivity of researchers than most organizations that sponsor or commission systematic reviews. In the Cochrane Collaboration, for example, two years normally elapse between researchers' posting a protocol for a review and its publication. EPCs complete DERP reviews in eight to ten months (although the governance can grant extensions of one to two months). Participating organizations receive drafts at the end of the seventh month, at the same time that DERP staff solicits external reviews. When several leaders of Cochrane told Helfand at a meeting in 2005 that such rapid production embarrassed them, he replied, "It's satisfying to do reviews when Mark Gibson does your marketing."[30]

A significant methodological innovation by DERP has been the routine involvement of people who have different priorities in devising the key questions to be addressed by each review. These questions define the drugs in the class, diseases affected by the drugs, populations and outcomes of interest, and whether any other types of studies than randomized controlled trials will be reviewed. In contrast, researchers have set the key questions for most published systematic reviews, sometimes consulting clinicians and, much less frequently, patients. An EPC researcher remarked in 2008 that both the governance and the EPC staff were "increasingly sophisticated about outcomes" when setting key questions.[31]

DERP determines key questions in what Gibson described as "an iterative process," which often takes several months. At the beginning of this process, he wrote, "interested parties exchange feedback in public meetings held in participating states and researchers and policymakers consult with one another directly."[32] Staff then posts draft questions on the Web and invites comments on them from the pharmaceutical industry, associations of health professionals, and advocacy groups.

DERP expanded the process for devising key questions in 2007 by establishing Clinical Advisory Groups. Each of these groups consists of three experts selected by the governance to discuss draft key questions in conference calls. Members of these groups must disclose conflicts of interest; but, such conflicts, like those disclosed by advisers to the federal Food and Drug Administration, do not disqualify them.

At the close of the comment period, the policymakers in the DERP governance and the EPC researchers discuss the draft questions and comments on them until they reach consensus. Helfand has had an important role in helping policymakers describe what they want to know. Gibson recalls that, in order to focus the questions, Helfand frequently asked members of the governance "what they might do with information they were seeking."[33]

Three "template key questions" evolved to guide members and researchers in planning and conducting reviews:

- What is the comparative efficacy (or effectiveness, if good studies are available) of drugs in a class in improving (name the outcome desired) for (name type of patients by symptoms, disease, etc.)?

- What are the comparative incidence and nature of adverse events . . . for patients being treated for (name the type of patient by symptoms, disease, etc.)?

- Are there subgroups of patients based on demographic characteristics (age, racial/ethnic groups, gender), other medications or co-morbidities (obesity, for example) for which one or more medications or preparations are more effective or are associated with fewer adverse effects?[34]

DERP staff acquires clinical evidence from drug manufacturers in order to insulate the EPC from potential interference. Staff also sends the key questions for each review to all manufacturers of pharmaceutical drugs in

North America; and special notification (with a return receipt) to those that sell a drug in the class being reviewed. DERP asks the manufacturers to submit, at their own expense, a dossier of evidence about the effectiveness of a drug according to a specified format. DERP only accepts information the companies permit it to disclose to the public; staff returns information marked confidential. EPC researchers evaluate the quality of this evidence, as well as evidence in articles and unpublished reports gathered from international databases of the results of clinical research; they also do "hand searches" of journals for relevant studies.

DERP modified what it requested from manufacturers as it tightened its standards of scientific rigor. By 2006, staff no longer invited manufacturers to submit subjective judgments about the comparative effectiveness of a drug. They had by then also ceased requesting results of the animal studies that preceded trials in humans. To ensure completeness in acquiring evidence, staff briefly asked manufacturers of generic drugs for information, but ceased when they received no responses. DERP also accommodated to requests from manufacturers to simplify the dossier process, most of them expressed during annual meetings with industry representatives that began in 2004.

Science and the politics of policymaking also converge in external review of draft reports. Staff notifies medical specialty societies and organizations that advocate for patients of the opportunity to comment on a draft. Alison Little, a physician who became director of DERP in 2007, recalled that the "volume of comments we get from anyone other than industry is very small."[35] Staff also sends drafts for review to experts in evaluating evidence and on pertinent clinical issues and to members of a Clinical Advisory Group. They post these reviews on the Web. DERP, like peer-reviewed journals, has rejected requests from the drug industry to identify the external reviewers of each report; like journals, it periodically posts lists of reviewers.

The minutes of the governance document the thoroughness of the process of review and revision. Staff brings to the governance comments by external reviewers and organizations that address significant issues. For example, an intense discussion about comments on a draft review of statins occurred on a conference call in September 2005:

> The report has been sent for new peer review [as a result of public comments]. Mark Helfand sent Pfizer a detailed response to their public comment. . . . EPC asked six reviewers and AHRQ has asked NIH to also review. To date, one [reviewer] said . . . name/affiliation could [not] be released. All [reviewers] rated the review as excellent.

The reviewer from AHRQ suggests Key Questions be changed to address individual variability. Participating Organizations should consider this. In addition, the issue of predicting response based on LDL response (this was formerly a Key Question) was also raised by the AHRQ reviewer. Helfand noted there is insufficient evidence. Helfand [also] noted that there have been changes made in the [draft review] to address these comments. A few more changes/additions need to be made. Then, Helfand recommend[ed] finalizing the [review] and releas[ing] it (and deal with NIH peer review as it comes).[36]

DERP's process of research, analysis, external review, and revision enables it to array information in a format that assists policymakers in making decisions. When Gibson summarized the results of twenty-nine reviews of drug classes and almost fifty updates completed by late 2007, he displayed them in five categories. Each category made explicit the strength of the evidence about the potential benefits of the drugs and policy to prefer drugs in each class:

- Good evidence, no significant differences [among competing drugs] (e.g., proton pump inhibitors)
- No good comparative evidence (e.g., opioid analgesics)
- Good evidence, marginal differences (e.g., triptans)
- Good evidence, significant clinical differences (e.g., beta blockers)
- Good evidence but with significant gaps (e.g., subpopulations)[37]

Arraying research findings in these categories clarifies policymakers' choices. It also enables them to predict which interest and advocacy groups their decisions will please, which groups they will disappoint, and how strongly disappointed groups will probably protest.

DERP AND THE PHARMACEUTICAL INDUSTRY

Categorizing research findings so that public benefits and political risks become transparent threatens the market share of many prescription drugs, and hence the revenues of pharmaceutical companies. Manufacturers had customarily marketed their drugs to state policymakers by lobbying officials who made coverage decisions (sometimes the lobbyists were former state policymakers), contributing to political campaigns, subsidizing selected nonprofit groups that advocate for patients (sometimes creating such groups), and providing rebates to states and PBMs under contract to them.

Because states spend billions of dollars for drugs, manufacturers had to cooperate with DERP. While cooperating, however, most of the companies and their surrogates challenged its methodology and the findings of its reports nationally and within states.[38]

Anti-DERP activity by the industry has been extensive. Articles challenging the methodology of DERP reviews are published in peer-reviewed journals. The authors of many of these articles work directly for pharmaceutical companies or consult with or receive grants from them. These articles are persuasive to clinicians who are inclined to be persuaded. A researcher at an EPC reported, for example, that a DERP review "caused internal problems at the University" because it was "not saying the right things" according to senior members of a clinical department.

Newsletters of health organizations and talks by experts paid by industry to meetings of physicians, pharmacists, and patient advocacy groups summarize anti-DERP articles in journals. The prose in newsletters and talks often duplicates the wording of letters complaining about DERP's methods and findings that leaders of advocacy groups, joined by some organizations of physicians and researchers, send to officials of state government and the federal Centers for Medicare and Medicaid. These groups also post their letters on the Web and distribute them by e-mail. An EPC researcher recalled that a pharmaceutical manufacturer and the National Alliance for the Mentally Ill, a national advocacy group that has affiliates in every state, inadvertently used identical words in criticizing a review.[39]

The industry has used two rhetorical strategies to attack DERP's credibility: attack the methodology of drug class reviews; and attack how the findings of reviews could be used. Articles and PowerPoint presentations critical of DERP's methodology usually acknowledge that systematic reviews advance knowledge about the effectiveness of interventions. But their authors frequently imply that the international standing of systematic reviews is no higher than that of other methodologies. Then the critics allege that reviews have serious methodological problems. These include variation in the quality of evidence in clinical trials, the absence of evidence from observational studies of outcomes, and the difficulty of addressing co-morbidities.

The critics' most frequent criticism of the methodology of reviews is a truism: that statistical inferences about a population do not apply to all the individuals within it, and especially not to underrepresented subpopulations such as children and members of minority groups. Many of them use this unassailable statement to justify covering any drug that is safe. In disparaging measures of the effects of drugs in populations, that is,

DERP's critics embrace a lower threshold for marketing a drug than the standards of the Food and Drug Administration, which require the demonstration of efficacy in populations as well as of safety.

Moreover, critics of DERP's methodology frequently read and quote selectively. For example, those who charge that systematic reviews ignore "scientifically valid [observational] research [on outcomes]" themselves ignore considerable evidence to the contrary. Fred Mosteller praised Iain Chalmers and his colleagues for using observational research as well as RCTs in the reviews included in the landmark volumes of *Effective Care in Pregnancy and Childbirth*.[40] Cochrane Collaboration Methods Groups routinely report new ways to grade the quality of evidence and to include observational and even qualitative research in reviews.[41] Similarly, many critics of DERP have quoted a warning about the limits of evidence-based health research in a classic article by David Sackett, a pioneer of the field. But they ignore Sackett's theme, which is the desirability of integrating rigorous research with clinical judgment. In the same article, however, Sackett also warns that "non-experimental approaches . . . routinely lead to false-positive conclusions about efficacy."[42]

Scientific judgment has sometimes prevailed over the industry's rhetoric of attack. For instance, a journal invited Gibson and Santa to reply to an article criticizing DERP's methods that it had accepted for publication. Three of the four authors of this article had disclosed to the journal that they were employed by or consulted to a pharmaceutical manufacturer. The editor sent Gibson's and Santa's reply to the authors and requested a rejoinder. They withdrew the paper.[43]

The second rhetorical strategy of DERP's industry critics is to describe the uses of systematic reviews in words that could mobilize physicians and patients to oppose decisions about coverage informed by them. These critics often use phrases introduced decades earlier, some of them identified in Chapter 2, in order to raise anxiety among physicians about the findings of research on health services. Some critics allege that Medicaid bureaucrats without clinical training use statistical inferences to contradict physicians' judgment and thus limit patients' freedom of choice. Dissident Canadian physicians, invited to Oregon by opponents of its PDL, said that systematic reviews were another unfortunate result of socialized medicine. Code phrases of more recent origin predict harm to poor people and especially members of minority groups covered by Medicaid because coverage policy informed by DERP reviews would allegedly deny them access to potentially beneficial drugs. Systematic reviews, other critics have said, also offered a rationalization for covert rationing in order to reduce costs.

Several implied that former Oregon officials wanted DERP to expand to other states the policy of overt rationing of services for Medicaid recipients they had introduced in the early 1990s.

The chairman of Pfizer until 2007, Henry McKinnell, gave speeches and interviews in which he sought to raise anxiety about the uses of systematic reviews. He insisted that policy "should allow doctors and patients to choose the best courses of care," but that PDLs offered less than the best. In April 2005, McKinnell told the *Medical Herald*, a newsletter, that policy informed by systematic reviews could harm African-Americans and Hispanics.[44] Employees of Pfizer regularly published criticism of the methods and findings of particular systematic reviews, including DERP's.

In 2005, McKinnell spoke at a meeting on global health policy, a subject on which he is a recognized expert. In a side conversation before the meeting, another participant asked his opinion about using systematic reviews to inform policy for covering drugs in low-income countries. McKinnell said that he had never heard the phrase systematic review.

Direct political action is considerably more dangerous than rhetoric for state policymakers and DERP. In 2006 and 2008, DERP staff asked participating organizations to describe how the industry and its surrogates challenged decisions about preferred drugs. Officials from eight states replied in writing, others orally. They reported that the most frequent activities were:

- Intervention in governors' offices by individual companies to request that drugs they manufactured be added to the preferred list

- Organized letter-writing by physicians to legislators on behalf of designating particular drugs as preferred

- Testimony by company representatives and their surrogates on behalf of preferring particular drugs at public meetings of committees that advise state agencies about what to include on the PDL

- Lobbying of legislators and officials of the executive branch by mental health advocacy groups to exclude drugs to treat mental illness from PDLs

- Lobbying of legislative minority caucuses to exclude from PDLs drugs to treat asthma as well as mental illness

- Lobbying by companies and their surrogates to weaken the criteria for requiring prior authorization; for instance, by loosening the definition of "clinical superiority," or by permitting physicians to prescribe drugs for which there is no evidence of superiority

- Lobbying to weaken PDLs by legislation prohibiting, for example, removing drugs after listing or requiring that at least two brand-name drugs be preferred

Only a few member states mentioned industry attempts to prevent their joining or continuing in DERP. However, Gibson has first-hand knowledge of four states that did not join DERP, for reasons that included opposition from the drug industry and its surrogates. The chief pharmacist in another state told him that the "industry is our friend."

Industry tactics sometimes exceed such routine lobbying. One state official reported that "[company name] had my personal physician, who is on its speakers list, call me to complain" about a DERP review. A lobbyist invited her husband to a golf event sponsored by the same company, and then asked, "What's your wife doing with [brand-name drug]?"

The history of the inception of the PDL in New York exemplifies the industry's influence and its limits. Richard Gottfried, chair of the Health Committee of the New York State Assembly recalled in 2009, that, in 2003, when he introduced legislation to create a PDL, he expected the "struggle would be to get the Republican Pataki Administration and state Senate majority to agree that the program could be effective . . . and to convince some Democrats in the Assembly majority (where the drug companies have considerable lobbying influence) that the consumer protections were strong enough."

During 2003 and early negotiations about the next state budget in 2004, Gottfried continued,

> intense drug company lobbying was convincing some Assembly Democrats that the PDL would block Medicaid recipients (especially Blacks and Hispanics) from getting the best drugs. A small number of legislators carried that message, sometimes tinged with racial rhetoric. Drug companies have persuasive lobbyists, and make extensive contributions to campaigns, community organizations and various disease advocacy groups. . . . The Pataki Administration did not believe a PDL would work with the consumer protections I wanted. . . . [Moreover,] opponents in the Assembly limited how far I could go without creating bitter division within the Democratic conference. The Assembly speaker concluded, correctly, that the negotiations could not reach agreement and he took the issue off the table.

By 2005, Gottfried had persuaded both the Pataki Administration and his Assembly colleagues that the bill creating the PDL included appropriate protection for consumers. The bill became law, covering enrollees in Medicaid and the Elderly Pharmaceutical Insurance Coverage (EPIC) program; and authorizing the state to join DERP. In 2008, the legislature extended PDL coverage to Family Health Plus, the state's Medicaid expansion program. Gottfried notes that since the inception of the PDL, "I have not had a single complaint about it from a constituent or health care provider, and none of my legislative colleagues have told me they have had any complaints."[45]

There is other evidence that lobbying by the industry can be neutralized. Several state medical societies support their state's membership in DERP. In some states the industry and its surrogates have not objected when laws prohibiting the inclusion of drugs for mental illness, AIDS/HIV, and cancer lapsed. Officials in several states report that representatives of manufacturers ask them to send new studies of their products to DERP.

Most important, the committees and officials that select preferred drugs for most of the PDLs established by 2008 continue to rely on independent research. "Overall, states reported relying on evidence-based research (comparative effectiveness reviews, research from peer-reviewed journals, etc.) more heavily than on supplemental rebate information when establishing coverage policy," a survey by the National Association of State Medicaid Directors (NASMD) found in 2007.[46]

REVISITING THE CAUSES OF CONVERGENCE
Persons

The causes of convergence, introduced in Chapter 1 and documented in Chapters 2 and 3, are abstractions that do not adequately convey the intellectual curiosity, energy, integrity, and courage of the public officials who have implemented and defended it. Abstractions also mask the anger, frustration, and fatigue as well as the satisfaction and sometimes joy that accompany immersion in the politics of making policy.

In order to explain the success of convergence to date, I focus first on particular policymakers and then, in the concluding section of the chapter, on evidence that the risks they took have been justified. Advances in research methods that had practical applications, the growing competence of state government, the increasing costs of health care, and the rising incidence and prevalence of chronic disease made convergence possible. Uncertain state revenue, the growing cost of pharmaceutical drugs, the inefficiency of health services, and the familiarity of senior state officials with the methods and uses of health services research made convergence feasible. Individual policymakers made convergence happen.

The daily experience of senior officials in most states early in this decade prepared them to consider new health policy if it could contain the growth of spending. States' revenue from taxes and fees began to fall during the first half of 2000 as a result of the recession. Revenue did not recover until several years after the official end of the recession in 2001. During the same years, the cost of pharmaceuticals was increasing. As a result of this financial situation, every official who participated in establishing PDLs and DERP had participated in decisions about which citizens would have less access to health services.

These officials knew a great deal about the citizens in their state whose suffering increased as their access to health care declined. Many of the people who lost all or some of their coverage under Medicaid had at least one serious chronic disease. Many were elderly. Many younger people affected by cuts in Medicaid budgets had disabling mental and physical conditions. Legislators who represented these citizens described the effects of their reduced access to care to their colleagues and to officials of the executive branch. Officials of both branches heard about the problems created by reduced budgets from representatives of hospital associations and community health centers and of groups that advocated on behalf of the elderly, racial and ethnic minorities, women, and persons with physical disabilities, mental illness, asthma, Alzheimer's disease, heart disease, and cancer. News media reported on people whose suffering increased as their access to health care diminished.

Officials of the legislative and executive branches of the states discussed falling revenues and rising drug costs at meetings with colleagues from other states, including meetings of the Reforming States Group (RSG). Meetings of the RSG are nonpartisan, include legislative and executive branch leaders, are limited to no more than forty participants, and are conducted under the famous Las Vegas advertising slogan, modified as "What is said here stays here."

RSG members also shared stories about the marketing, pricing, and political and legal activities of the pharmaceutical industry. I reported several of James Haveman's stories about Michigan in Chapter 1. RSG members also followed a developing story about a lawsuit by the industry against Kevin Concannon, then the secretary of health and human services in Maine.

A 2000 statute created Maine Rx, a program to lower the price of prescription drugs for every resident of the state to the price charged to persons eligible for Medicaid. Federal law required manufacturers to discount, through rebates to the state, the price of drugs for Medicaid recipients by 20–25 percent below the retail price. The state now mandated the same discount for other citizens. The state also required that physicians request prior authorization to prescribe drugs from manufacturers that refused to offer this discount. The pharmaceutical industry claimed in its lawsuit that Maine Rx interfered with interstate commerce and violated federal Medicaid law by subsidizing health services for persons who were not medically indigent.[47]

The U.S. Supreme Court eventually upheld Maine's law in the case that began as *PhRMA v. Concannon*. RSG members relished Concannon's anecdotes about the case as it moved through federal courts. They particularly enjoyed his descriptions of courtroom confrontations between the two young assistant attorneys general who represented the state and the more numerous, more highly compensated, and better-dressed lawyers for the drug industry, who included the future Chief Justice John Roberts.

A growing number of RSG members had, moreover, first-hand experience of the methods and uses of systematic reviews and had worked with researchers who conducted them. Each year beginning in 1999, Lee Greenfield, a Minnesota policymaker who was a founder of the RSG and an early proponent of systematic reviews, recruited eight colleagues to participate in a five-day interactive workshop on the methods of evidence-based health research. By 2008, policymakers from more than thirty jurisdictions in the United States and Canada had participated in the workshop, which was then an annual event. A legislator told Greenfield after one workshop, "I can't wait for someone to bring a phony study before my committee." Another legislator asked to attend for a second time, "because it has changed how I think about all policy, not just health policy."[48]

In the fall of 2002, RSG members discussed the collaboration among Oregon, Idaho, and Washington to produce systematic reviews of drug classes. Mark Gibson, then a co-chair of the RSG, described the project to RSG members from across the country at three meetings.

Before each of the RSG's annual regional meetings in 2003, Greenfield and colleagues who had attended the five-day workshop led a half-day session to introduce other RSG members to evidence-based health research. They invited leading trialists and systematic reviewers from the United States and Canada to describe the techniques of critical appraisal, particularly how to identify common types of bias in primary studies. These researchers then provided technical assistance to breakout groups in which participants appraised an RCT and then a systematic review. Approximately

100 policymakers from the legislative and executive branches participated in these meetings.[49]

Many people in state government have contributed to establishing PDLs and DERP. RSG members in particular endorsed DERP from the outset, brought some of their states into the collaboration, and helped repel attacks on PDLs and on DERP by the pharmaceutical industry and its surrogates. The personal and professional commitment of members of the DERP governance has made it an organization that enables states to spend more efficiently for beneficial drugs.

Mark Gibson and John Kitzhaber made unique contributions to DERP's prominence as an agent of convergence. Colleagues for many years in and out of government, they are committed to improving health through policy that is informed by the best available evidence. As governor of Oregon, Kitzhaber created one of the first PDLs and commissioned the first systematic reviews to inform drug coverage for Medicaid. Out of office as a result of term limits at the end of 2002, he encouraged and inspired members of the DERP governance and staff in meetings and defended convergence in speeches and interviews.

Gibson has traveled the country to establish and maintain support for DERP in state government and to debate its critics. When DERP began Gibson was an able and experienced analyst and author of policy, an accomplished political strategist, and an effective public spokesman. Leading DERP, he also became an adroit manager of the production and dissemination of systematic reviews and a skilled polemicist in the United States and abroad on behalf of good science and its application to policy.

Major news media have assisted state officials in defending PDLs and DERP by covering convergence accurately and frequently. Media coverage was most intense in the fall 2004, when Merck recalled the painkiller Vioxx because of evidence of its adverse effects. Newspapers and television stations across the country ran an Associated Press story in November of that year reporting that officials in Oregon, Washington State, and Idaho had made public a systematic review in 2002 that called attention to these adverse effects. According to the story, Oregon and Washington had removed Vioxx from their lists of preferred drugs. The story also quoted a member of the DERP governance: "Missouri applied the Vioxx warning to a computer program that in fewer than three seconds judges whether the state should pay for prescriptions."[50] In other stories in the same months, the *New York Times* and the *Wall Street Journal* also credited DERP with an early warning on Vioxx.[51] The *Washington Post* and the *Boston Globe* ran stories that related the finding of adverse effects from

Vioxx to a new project of Consumers' Union to bring the findings of DERP reviews to the general public.[52]

A columnist for the *Wall Street Journal* who was also Washington Bureau Chief for MSNBC sharply rejected the pharmaceutical industry's attacks on DERP. In November 2004, under the headline "Trade Group's Fight Against Drug Review is Self-Defeating," Alan Murray wrote, "If drug companies honestly think the Oregon project isn't the best source of information, then they should take the lead in coming up with alternatives." He defended drug class reviews as good science and as the basis for proper economic evaluation.[53]

DERP continues to gain support despite the persistence of its critics. Officials of the Veteran's Administration use DERP reviews to inform decisions about drug coverage. The federal Agency for Healthcare Research and Quality (AHRQ) funds the Center for Evidence-based Policy, DERP's parent organization, to assist in "stakeholder outreach" in conducting systematic reviews of the comparative effectiveness of interventions. The newsletter of the American Academy of Child and Adolescent Psychiatry described DERP as the "leading U.S. drug-assessment initiative."[54]

Some advocates of legislation initially introduced in Congress in 2007 and enacted in 2009 to create a national program of research to compare the effectiveness of health services (see Chapter 5 for more on comparative effectiveness research) consider DERP to be what U.S. Senator Ron Wyden (D-Ore.) and Ezekiel Emanuel, then of the National Institutes of Health and now on the White House staff, called a "useful model."[55] Wyden and Emanuel, however, misconstrued DERP as a "collaboration of public and private organizations" that includes states. However, DERP is governed and sustained by states and a Canadian intergovernmental agency; its credibility is based on holding private organizations, especially drug manufacturers and their surrogates, at arm's length.

DERP is, moreover, expanding the scope of its work in ways that are likely to cause additional health sector interest groups to express consternation at being held at arm's length. In 2008, its governance began to plan a third three-year cycle. Work under discussion for this cycle includes commissioning more reviews on the full range of treatments for specific diseases rather than on drug classes alone, comparison among classes, and reviewing combination drugs and the effectiveness of biologicals and orphan drugs.

DERP's reviews are also informing drug purchasing decisions by individual consumers. In testimony before the Committee on Ways and Means of the U.S. House of Representatives in 2007, Gail Shearer of

Consumers' Union reported on the results of DERP reviews reformatted for its publication *Consumer Reports Best Buy Drugs*®. Enrollees in Medicare Part D who chose preferred drugs "in five leading categories . . . can save up to $5,000 a year," she said. Moreover, "those switching to the preferred drug in just one drug category can typically save more than enough to cover the cost of their Part D premium."[56]

DERP reviews reported in *Best Buy Drugs* helped to generate support for legislation to create a federal program of comparative effectiveness research. A member of the U.S. Senate health staff reported early in 2009, when passage of the legislation was still uncertain, that "Consumer Report's *Best Buy* work has done an awful lot to legitimize comparative effectiveness here in DC."

Building on the success of DERP, the Center for Evidence-based Policy collaborated with states beginning in 2006 to organize a new program, Medicaid Evidence-based Decision Making (MED). This program conducts reviews and technology assessments for collaborating states across the range of interventions covered by Medicaid. Because timeliness often matters in making decisions about coverage, MED's staff and external researchers produces rapid analyses as well as more extensive evidence reviews. The states collaborating in MED have, for the first time, research and development capacity similar to that of Kaiser Permanente, the Veterans Health Administration, and other integrated delivery systems in the United States, and to that of governments in countries that have universal coverage.

Cost Savings and Quality Improvement

Convergence occurred and has expanded because it has practical value for policymakers. Each policymaker who supports it continuously calculates its benefits and costs. Each of them will support convergence as long as he or she has persuasive evidence that it benefits consumers and contains the growth of the cost of public sector health coverage without subjecting them to career-threatening political risks. Evidence that political risks have been contained is often indirect. In one state in 2008, for example, "PhRMA [Pharmaceutical Research and Manufacturers of America] couldn't find a sponsor" for legislation to weaken the extent to which systematic reviews could inform decisions about the PDL.

Evidence that PDLs contain costs is persuasive. Researchers reported in a journal article in 2006 that Medicaid pharmacy costs in Oregon decreased 9.1 percent under the initial policy that permitted physicians to override the preferred drug themselves; and 17.7 percent when the state imposed a "soft pre-authorization policy."[57] Three other states that are members of DERP reported savings that by 2008 ranged from approximately $1 to $82 per enrollee; total dollars saved in these states were reported to be $1.3, $9 and $80 million.[58] Another state reported that the "PDL has returned roughly 5 percent of our drug spending in supplemental rebates."

Many anecdotes suggest that savings also occurred in other states that established PDLs that are informed by independent research. The major cause of savings, a member of the DERP governance said, is that "moving market share is the hammer." John Santa recalled his surprise when several states made Nexium, a prescription drug, a preferred proton pump inhibitor. DERP's review had found that the less expensive Prilosec, which is available without a prescription, was as effective as Nexium. He soon learned the reason: "Astra-Zenica had dropped the price of Nexium below the price of Prilosec."[59]

These reports of savings understate the effects of PDLs on cost. "Everyone measures market share and savings," a member of the DERP governance said. But Medicaid agencies are reluctant to report savings to the legislature in order to prevent, as another member said, being told "that was great now do more" or to have the savings applied to offset appropriations. As a result, most Medicaid programs report savings in general terms and sometimes apply them to "justify other programs as budget neutral," a member said. Moreover, pharmaceutical manufacturers are intensely aware of the savings. In one state, a lobbyist told the Medicaid director, "You're balancing your budget on PhRMA's back. The director replied, "Yes, we are."

DERP member states also report improvements in the quality of care because PDLs shift market share toward more effective drugs. A member of the governance reported that for some drugs, market share had moved in 80–90 percent of claims. Officials in another state reported a shift of market share from 2.64 percent to 84 percent for the preferred drug in one class, and from 25 percent to 90 percent in another, even though physicians could "switch to a non-preferred agent after trial with a preferred agent." The same state reported additional quality improvement because the "move to the PDL also included clinical criteria" developed with physicians that "prevented therapeutic duplication, [and] established minimum and maximum . . . doses."

Some states have documented that quality improvement is linked to cost savings. The Idaho Medicaid program, for example, calculated savings of $340,000 during the first six months after it implemented the findings of a DERP review of newer anti-convulsant drugs in 2005. Savings had increased to $1,440,213 by November 2007. An Idaho official also reported "positive outcomes and no negative outcomes," as well as a significant reduction in claims per month (about 7 percent over two years) as a result of the agency's efforts to discourage inappropriate prescribing.[60]

In another state, mental health lobbyists and advocates had predicted that patients would be harmed if the PDL applied the findings of DERP's review of atypical anti-psychotic drugs. Research commissioned by the state found, a DERP governance member said, that "we didn't cause more admissions through emergency rooms or more crisis situations." On the contrary, "outpatient visits increased, which is what we wanted so that patients' regimens could be stabilized." Even the advocates agreed that the "uptake in output was a positive sign."

States and therefore taxpayers earn substantial returns on the cost of DERP. Through its first five years of activity, the collaborating states together spent approximately $6 million dollars to sustain DERP, approximately half of that total coming from federal matching funds. In 2005 alone, in contrast, state and local government spent more than $21.7 billion for prescription drugs.[61]

Despite considerable evidence of success, however, the convergence of research and policymaking for health in states is fragile. The survival of DERP and the widespread use of its reviews is proof of the viability of convergence as a concept. But proof of a concept is not proof that it is sustainable.

The fragility of convergence has several causes. Perhaps most important, state policymakers who initiate, manage, and support convergence are still outliers among their peers; and an increasing number no longer hold office. Another significant cause of fragility is a limited supply of health services researchers who work effectively where science and governance converge. A third source of fragility is the potential for attracting new antagonists—the medical device industry, for example—if the scope of convergence expands.

Convergence is fragile even though support for it is increasing. The next chapter assesses the political prospects of the convergence of independent research and health policy.

5. Can Convergence Be Sustained?

The underlying causes of the convergence of research and health policy-making described earlier in this book remain powerful. Research on the effectiveness and comparative effectiveness of health services is expanding in scope, scale and persuasiveness. Demand is growing—from state and federal policymakers, large corporate purchasers of care, health insurance plans and provider systems—for reliable evidence about effectiveness and quality. Policymakers are intent on containing the growth of spending for health care. The burden of chronic disease increases inexorably.

Significant potential causes of greater convergence were emerging as this book went into production. The national economic stimulus program (the American Recovery and Reinvestment Act of 2009, or ARRA) includes $1.1 billion for research on the comparative effectiveness of health services (CER). The acting director of the National Institutes of Health (NIH) announced that additional appropriations to his agency under the act would be used for CER. The high priority accorded to increased access to health care by the Obama administration and leading congressional Democrats was increasing the urgency of improving quality and efficiency in ways that contained the rate of growth in health care costs.

Evidence of successful convergence also contributes to its sustainability. Articles in peer-reviewed journals report beneficial effects and sometimes cost savings when research on effectiveness informs policy and improves the quality of clinical practice. Much of this literature evaluates demonstration projects. But the achievements of DERP and evidence from the Veterans Administration, Kaiser Permanente and other organizations in the United States and other countries suggests that convergence can be sustained in making decisions about clinical policy and translating that policy into practice.

Convergence threatens powerful individuals and interests, however. Although some organizations that educate, train, license, certify, and represent physicians have endorsed convergence, many physicians worry that it threatens their clinical autonomy. Senior executives of a few firms that manufacture pharmaceuticals acknowledge that independent systematic reviews of effectiveness and comparative effectiveness have become part of their regulatory environment. But other employees of the industry and their surrogates continue to criticize the methodology of systematic reviews and insist that states are using them to justify covering the cheapest drugs; and that the federal government may do so in the future. Many advocates for persons suffering particular diseases or chronic pain, and physicians associated with them, continue to demand coverage for every drug or procedure that regulators deem to be safe and that could be effective.

Politics is determining the sustainability of convergence. In politics as in securities markets, past performance does not predict future events; but it may be instructive. The politics of achieving the limited success of convergence in American states has had five attributes:

- Policymakers understood the methods and potential uses of independent research on the effectiveness of health services
- Policymakers had access to an increasingly comprehensive array of potentially useful research results
- Trusted intermediaries assisted policymakers and researchers in understanding methodology and assessing the potential uses of research findings
- Researchers who had appropriate knowledge, communication skills, freedom from conflicts of interest and a commitment to convergence conducted evidence reviews in order to inform policymaking
- Policymakers who initiated and defended convergence had sufficient support from major print and electronic media, some interest and advocacy groups, and voters to overcome or neutralize organized antagonism to it

In this chapter I assess opportunities and problems associated with each of these attributes of the politics of successful convergence. I do so in order to help persons who believe that the convergence of research with policymaking for health is in the public interest to prepare for the contingencies ahead. I offer no recommendations, because recommendations that are not specific to particular situations are hardly ever useful to policymakers.

UNDERSTANDING RESEARCH ON EFFECTIVENESS

An important attribute of the convergence described in this book has been that policymakers who were influential among their peers understood the methods, findings and potential uses of rigorous, independent research on the effectiveness of health services. These methods and findings met the criteria they use to assess information.

Policymakers are wary of acting on information they do not understand and trust. Acting on information that is biased or inaccurate could harm their constituents and their careers. Most policymakers learn early in their public lives that they can assess the potential benefits and harms from acting on new information only when they trust it and trust its source.

Most health policymakers routinely receive information and advice from sources who claim that it is scientific. This information is frequently flawed by one or more of the systematic errors that researchers call bias. It is, moreover, often flawed by the nonscientific form of bias that is colloquially called spin. When policymakers discover that information is biased, the advocates and experts who gave it to them frequently defend themselves with platitudes about the uncertainty of science and their eagerness to help patients. The subtext of many health researchers in testimony at legislative hearings or in interviews with the media is that, although science is uncertain, policymakers should assume the risks of failed treatments and wasted resources on behalf of patients and those who love them.

Policymakers are accountable for their decisions, either directly to voters or to the officials of general government who appoint and confirm them. Most policymakers learn which experts they can trust to offer information that is consistently valid and reliable. They particularly appreciate experts who are discreet, and who understand that media coverage, while it is essential for policymakers, is merely satisfying and sometimes lucrative for experts.

Policymakers must acquire and act promptly on information about many issues. They analyze this information under the stress of deadlines, media coverage, importuning by lobbyists and advocates, and requests from voters. Because they are extremely busy, they prefer to receive summaries of research results and the recommendations based on them before they budget time to assess their credibility and salience and the feasibility of applying them to policy. Once they decide to assess a research result as a potential basis for policy, however, they insist on understanding as completely as possible whether they should trust it and for whom it is controversial.

These generalizations about policymakers and information differ from the views of many of the academics who study the dissemination of research. According to many articles about dissemination, a field recently renamed "knowledge transfer and exchange" (KTE), policymakers have little interest in or patience with research. As Jonathan Lomas, a founder of KTE in Canada, who has influenced its development in other countries wrote in 2007, policymakers "tend to see research as a product they can purchase from the local knowledge store."[1] To provide this information, adherents of KTE created a new profession in the 1990s; knowledge brokers whose expertise is in communications rather than research. These brokers convert findings from research into words and images that they hope can be "transferred" and applied. They are usually not concerned about policymakers' understanding and appreciation of research methods.

Theorists and advocates of KTE have evaluated its effectiveness and published their findings. Most of this research has been financed by public agencies and philanthropic organizations that fund research and that, therefore, have an incentive to demonstrate the usefulness of work they support. Almost all of these studies are based on written questionnaires and structured interviews rather than on direct observation of policymaking. The investigators sometimes ask policymakers and members of their staff what information from research they have used, what they want in the future, and what impedes their use of research findings. They rarely ask them to describe how they do their work and how the quality of information from research and other sources affects that work.[2]

Other studies ignore policymakers entirely. The authors of one frequently cited study, for example, did not interview elected officials because, the lead author told me, he and his colleagues assumed that civil servants are the most influential consumers of research that is relevant to policy for population health.[3] Another study described the role of research in policymaking entirely from the point of view of external "policy advisers."[4]

The assumption that policymakers are poor consumers of research causes KTE experts to ignore the complicated, often chaotic, processes by which policymakers are "staffed." Because these processes are intense, the verb "to staff" conveys strong feelings about integrity, loyalty, and accuracy when used to describe relationships between policymakers and their staff, as well as among staff members. Policymakers consume research when they trust its source, and their trust is strongest when it comes from knowledgeable staff or experts who have earned recognition as surrogate staff. They expect staff and surrogate staff to protect them against unpleasant surprises such as attacks on the accuracy of information they use and the independence of the sources of that information. Generalists serving as knowledge brokers rarely have sufficient knowledge to do this.

Unsurprisingly, most research on KTE has not demonstrated that it is effective, despite what evaluators of health services would call its "sponsorship bias." A systematic review published in 2007 found no evidence that KTE programs increase health policymakers' use of research to inform their decisions.[5] Similarly, in an article on "indifference to research-based evidence," Steven Lewis, a Canadian policy adviser and researcher, faulted KTE advocates for offering evidence as a "toolbox" rather than presenting research methods as potentially useful "habits of mind."[6]

Contrary to what the literature on KTE suggests, many policymakers are sympathetic to methodology for evaluating the effectiveness of health services because of their experience of politics. The fundamental principles of this methodology are that populations are the appropriate unit of analysis and that study designs should prevent bias. All policymakers serve defined populations. Legislators serve at their pleasure. Policymakers, moreover, are expert consumers of bias in the form of false or, more often, incomplete information or, especially in health affairs, wishful thinking by advocates and overly enthusiastic academic investigators.

Evidence-based health research can both augment and contradict anecdotal evidence. Policymakers are sensitive to the power of anecdotes. I have been quoted in various publications (and on a T-shirt) as saying that the "plural of anecdote is policy." Everyone in politics knows the constructive as well as the destructive power of stories—that "narrative matters," in a phrase devised by Fitzhugh Mullan, an author, physician, and former policymaker.[7] Elected officials and their staff frequently hear affecting anecdotes from voters seeking access to care and changes in policy. They also know first-hand that lobbyists and advocacy groups amplify the significance of anecdotes and impute opinions about them to voters; and that opinions about anecdotes in editorials and on talk shows inform but do not necessarily represent public opinion.

Policymakers' attentiveness to public opinion also makes them informed consumers of research methods that reduce systematic bias. Every elected official is a student of political polls. Each of them knows about sampling frames and margins of error and that polling results are affected by how questions are phrased, the order in which they are asked, and who asks them. For some of the policymakers who helped establish DERP the words bias and confidence had roughly similar operational definitions in both politics and statistics.

In each of the previous chapters I described meetings in which policymakers in state government learned about the methods and uses of evidence-based health research. In conversations following these meetings, many policymakers drew an analogy between their population-based profession and population-based research on the effectiveness of health services.

Convergence in state government could be sustained if legislative leaders and senior officials of the executive branch—those defined as "general government" in Chapter 3—remain familiar with the evolving methods and uses of evidence-based health research. Only general government can protect convergence from its detractors and expand its scope by mobilizing public opinion as well as allies across political parties and agencies of government.

But many current leaders of general government may not continue to follow advances in the methods of research that made convergence possible. A growing number of the policymakers who overcame the initial resistance to convergence among interest and advocacy groups are no longer in office as a result of term limits, job changes, the election of new governors, and retirement. The Reforming States Group continues to recruit and inform new members; but its outreach may not be sufficient to sustain convergence.

Convergence can only be sustained and extended if policymakers are aware of innovation in research methods and new findings from applying them. Methods of evaluating effectiveness are evolving rapidly. For example, researchers and their funders are devising and promoting substitutes for expensive and lengthy randomized controlled trials (RCTs) and systematic reviews. Such alternative methods include simulations, data-mining in electronic health records, and creating registries of patients who have particular conditions or receive particular interventions and become subjects in "practical trials."[8] Each of these alternative methods has strengths and weaknesses; each is also a source of income or potential income for researchers and research firms.

Reduced attention to emerging methods of research among leaders of general government could be an unintended consequence of the relative success of convergence. Leaders in general government are preoccupied with new issues and crises. In the states where convergence is occurring, these leaders have delegated to specialized government the task of managing the processes through which the best available evidence informs decisions about coverage. Most members of the governance of DERP and MED and the staff of state PDLs are officials of specialized government. They cannot routinely command the time and attention of general government.

ACCESS TO USEFUL RESEARCH RESULTS

During most of the history presented in Chapters 2 and 3, the convergence of science and governance in policymaking for health was an attractive, but rarely achieved, goal for many researchers and some policymakers. Convergence became practicable during the 1990s because researchers had developed persuasive methods for evaluating the effectiveness of health services and were applying them in fair tests of thousands of interventions. In 1983, in contrast, the U.S. Congress Office of Technology Assessment had documented the relative underfunding and underutilization of randomized controlled trials (RCTs) to evaluate the effectiveness of health services.[9] Several years earlier, making an ironical point to colleagues on the staff of a federal agency, I suggested that the cost of health services could be reduced if providers were reimbursed only for interventions that had been found to be effective by RCTs. This suggestion is no longer so ironical.

By the mid-1990s, thousands of researchers all over the world were evaluating interventions in studies that met high standards for both rigor and for disclosing potential conflicts of interest. Primary studies evaluated the outcomes of health interventions using a variety of experimental, quasi-experimental and observational methods. Systematic reviews made possible the convergence of research and policymaking for health by making the best evidence accessible and persuasive. The publication of *Effective Care in Pregnancy and Childbirth* at the beginning of the decade demonstrated the feasibility of evaluating interventions across an entire field of health care.[10] By the end of the 1990s, just over a thousand interventions to prevent, diagnose, treat, and manage an enormous variety of conditions had been evaluated in systematic reviews. In 2002, leaders of the Cochrane Collaboration told the officials who participated in its Funders and Users Forum that approximately 10,000 reviews would be required to evaluate every current intervention. By then several thousand new and updated reviews were being published each year.

Government subsidy to conduct systematic reviews increased during the 1990s in response to the establishment of the Cochrane Collaboration and new policy for PDLs in Australia, Canada, and New Zealand. The government of the United Kingdom became the largest funder of Cochrane reviews. Since 1999, moreover, the National Institute for Clinical Excellence (later Health and Clinical Excellence but still using NICE as its acronym) in that country has conducted reviews and issued "guidance" to policymakers and providers. Public agencies in Australia, Canada, New Zealand, and the Nordic countries commission Cochrane reviews. Although spending for systematic reviews in the United States began to increase substantially in the late 1990s, it did not match spending by these countries on a per capita basis until, as a result of the ARRA of 2009, it vastly exceeded it.

Despite increased funding, researchers in most countries say that they need more support for full-time staff (which they call infrastructure) that can produce high-quality evidence reviews on demand. Very few organizations have research teams whose primary job is producing reviews. Most researchers supplement commissions for evidence reviews, and especially for systematic reviews, with funds from university teaching and service budgets, grants for other purposes, and overhead from grants and contracts.

Even more important, there is frequently insufficient primary research to answer the policy questions systematic reviews could address.[11] Primary research, especially RCTs, requires considerable lead time and more funding than has been available. In the absence of primary research, systematic reviews can only discover gaps in knowledge and summarize the best available evidence.

Independent research evaluating health services, both primary studies and evidence reviews, has had considerably lower priority for funding than investigator-initiated research on what the NIH describes in its mission statement as the "causes, diagnosis, prevention and cure of human disease."[12] Agencies that are counterparts of the NIH in other countries have also been reluctant to finance evidence reviews. The agencies that fund biomedical research in every country prefer to invest in hypotheses that are proposed by investigators and reviewed by committees of peers for plausibility, potential significance, and likelihood to be tested appropriately. A recent recommendation by Iain Chalmers and colleagues that applicants to these organizations for research grants submit systematic reviews as evidence of the significance of the work they propose is as ironical as my suggestion thirty years ago that only interventions of proven effectiveness should be reimbursed.[13]

Many researchers, moreover, continue to disregard systematic reviews. Mike Clarke, Sally Hopewell, and Chalmers reported in 2007, for example, that "there is no evidence of progress between 1997 and 2005 in the proportion of reports of trials published in general medical journals which discussed new results within the context of up-to-date systematic reviews of relevant evidence from other controlled trials."[14]

Nevertheless, funding to conduct more evidence reviews and to update them is increasing because more policymakers are finding them useful. Reviews have the potential to change the politics of policymaking. Few policymakers are comfortable taking sides among experts on biomedical science, especially those who receive funding for research, consultation, or both from well-financed interest and advocacy groups. State-of-the-art systematic reviews can often obviate the need to take sides.

Legislators have been embarrassed when they adjudicated among experts in response to lobbying, advocacy, and public hearings. A recent book describes how legislatures in eleven states in the mid-1990s mandated a procedure called Autologous Bone Marrow Transplantation (ABMT) for women with breast cancer. These mandates were the result of intense advocacy by surgeons, women's health organizations, and individual patients with breast cancer and their families. Contrary to this advocacy, independent reviews by highly reputed technology assessment organizations demonstrated that ABMT decreased survival time, lowered the quality of life, and increased expense.

In the absence of a relatively insulated governmental locus for convergence, these reviews had no influence on policy. However, the reviews and new clinical trials eventually persuaded surgeons to abandon ABMT. In addition, an audit found that an investigator had falsified the data in a clinical trial on which surgeons and other advocates had relied.[15]

The ABMT story is a particularly harsh example of harm to patients and unnecessary spending as a result of policymaking by advocacy in the absence of governance that is informed by high-quality systematic reviews. Such reviews are what the authors of a book about their methodology call "a quantum leap" in evaluating health services. They meet high standards for framing questions, identifying relevant studies, appraising their quality, summarizing the evidence, and interpreting the findings.[16] Authors of reviews of the highest quality are, moreover, free of conflicts of interest as a result of funding by manufacturers of drugs and devices.

TRUSTED INTERMEDIARIES

Policymakers frequently rely on intermediaries to help them understand the methods and potential uses of research on health services. Chapters 1 and 3 have described the intermediary role of staff and advisers to the User Liaison Program (ULP) of the federal agency that is now the Agency for

Healthcare Research and Quality (AHRQ). Much of what ULP accomplished happened outside formal presentations and facilitated group discussion. Moreover, state officials who advised the ULP also attended its meetings and talked informally with participants, some of whom subsequently sought their advice on policy. Such active intermediaries included Mark Gibson, Lee Greenfield, Michigan State Representative David Hollister, and Iowa Senator Charles Bruner.

These intermediaries enhanced the relevance and clarity of researchers' presentations during pre-meeting rehearsals. Few researchers had experienced an appropriations chair (Hollister) interrupting their lecture to ask, "Excuse me doctor, but so what?"

Since the early 1990s, a growing number of public officials have become effective intermediaries between researchers and their colleagues. Bob Nakagawa of British Columbia has been an adviser on policy for pharmaceutical drugs to colleagues in Canada, the United States, and China, among other countries. Anne McFarlane, another Canadian, has been an intermediary in Canada, the United States, and other countries, while serving as a policymaker in provincial government and for an intergovernmental agency. Chris Henshall, Kent Woods, and Ron Stamp were effective intermediaries as officials of the Department of Health for England; as was Peter Donnelly, former deputy chief medical officer for the National Health Service in Scotland. Carolyn Clancy, director of AHRQ, and members of her staff are effective intermediaries in the United States.

The Milbank Memorial Fund has accorded priority to being an intermediary between policymakers and health researchers since 1990, resuming a role it had in the first three decades of the twentieth century. As president of the Fund, I joined Iain Chalmers in meetings with officials of the National Health Service about the relevance of systematic reviews for policy and practice in 1991 and led a workshop on how systematic reviews could inform policy at the second meeting of the Cochrane Collaboration in 1994. The Fund commissioned articles in 1991 (published in the *Milbank Quarterly* in 1993) on how systematic reviews could inform policy in Canada, the United Kingdom, and the United States.[17] In 1995, Lee Greenfield, Sheldon Greenfield a researcher at Tufts University (and no relation to Lee), Paul Cleary, a researcher at the Harvard Medical School, and B. D. Collen, a columnist for *Newsday*, convened researchers and state officials to review drafts of a report on the methods of research evaluating the outcomes of health care.[18] Andrew Oxman of Norway and the Cochrane Collaboration and Lee Greenfield assembled a textbook for policymakers attending the workshops on research methods described in Chapter 4. In

2000, the Fund assisted the Cochrane Collaboration in preparing a business plan in order to attract additional funding to support infrastructure for preparing systematic reviews. Between 2000 and 2005, the Fund and Cochrane leaders convened an annual forum of research funders and users from fifteen countries.

The Fund also assisted the Reforming States Group (RSG) in making its essential contributions to convergence. Since the inception of the RSG in 1991, members have set its agenda, led its projects, and invited colleagues, initially from other states, and then from other countries, to join them. Staff of the Fund provided logistical and editorial support and, when invited, technical assistance on issues of research and policy.

The Milbank Memorial Fund continues to be an intermediary under Carmen Hooker Odom, who became its president at the end of 2007. Hooker Odom was a legislative leader in Massachusetts and then secretary of the Department of Health and Human Services in North Carolina. She was for many years a member of the Steering Committee of the RSG.

A few other endowed foundations share the Fund's mission of responsiveness to policymakers. These include the California Health Care Foundation, the New York Health Foundation, the Canadian Foundation for Health Services Research and, in the United Kingdom, the Nuffield Trust and the Health Foundation.

The federal Centers for Medicare and Medicaid Services (CMS) has had a limited role in convergence in the states. The regulatory and funding authority of CMS is frequently a source of tension and often conflict with states. Nevertheless, CMS has permitted states' to use federal matching funds to finance DERP and MED.

The transfer of prescription drug coverage for persons dually eligible for Medicare and Medicaid from the states to the federal government in 2004 reduced the number of patients who benefit from convergence. Coverage decisions by the private insurers who offer the Medicare drug benefit under regulations issued by CMS are usually made on the basis of less rigorous evidence than state PDLs demand. Under the "clawback" provision of the Medicare Modernization Act of 2003, moreover, the states still pay a substantial portion of the cost of this coverage.

CMS is, however, helping to legitimize the convergence of science and governance in decisions about coverage for procedures and medical devices for which evidence of effectiveness is promising but inconclusive. Its program of "conditional coverage with evidence development" permits physicians to prescribe such intervention while participating in practice-based clinical trials.[19]

The potential federal role in convergence changed substantially early in 2009 when Congress appropriated $1.1 billion to evaluate the comparative effectiveness of health services. Support had been growing for comparative effectiveness research since Congress included a small appropriation for the Agency for Healthcare Research and Quality to initiate a program in the Medicare Modernization Act. Members of Congress introduced legislation to authorize a considerably larger program in 2007. The Congressional Budget Office reported in 2007 that conducting and applying research on comparative effectiveness could contribute to the efficiency of federal health spending, which, it argued, is increasing mainly as a result of the introduction of new technology.[20] Policy journals and newspapers published numerous articles describing the potential benefits of such a program and recommending ways to govern and finance it. A roundtable convened by the Institute of Medicine (IOM) has, since 2006, explored the prospects of a national comparative effectiveness program with leaders of medicine, hospitals and health systems, health plans and insurers, and the pharmaceutical industry.[21] An IOM report early in 2008, *Knowing What Works in Health Care*, recommended increased federal spending for comparative effectiveness research and systematic reviews.[22]

The economic stimulus legislation of 2009 appropriated funds for research on comparative effectiveness to AHRQ ($300 million), NIH ($400 million) and the secretary of health and human services ($400 million). It also provided for a contract to the IOM to develop recommendations for national priorities for the new research and established a fifteen-member Federal Coordinating Council for Comparative Effectiveness Research. Congress prohibited the council from establishing clinical guidelines or "mandat[ing] coverage, reimbursement or other policies for any public or private payer."[23] This prohibition responded to criticism of the new program by lobbyists for manufacturers of pharmaceutical drugs and medical devices and their surrogates, especially among advocates on behalf of persons with particular diseases. These lobbyists and advocates employed arguments similar to those they directed against Drug Effectiveness Review Program (DERP) reviews and state policy decisions on drug coverage. They complained, for instance, that the new research could lead to rationing care on the basis of cost. Moreover, according to W. J. (Billy) Tauzin, president of the leading pharmaceutical trade association and a former member of Congress, "Our medicines very often work better on some people than on other people." Coverage of criticism of the program by lobbyists and advocates in leading news outlets referred to the achievements of state drug coverage programs using research by DERP.[24]

The new program will be a year old when this book is published. By then it may not yet be clear precisely how comparative effectiveness research will inform coverage by public and private purchasers, how successful interest groups and advocates will be in compromising the independence of the research, and the extent to which the new federal funds will crowd out independent research sponsored by states.

RESEARCHERS WHO CAN INFORM POLICYMAKING

Sustaining convergence, especially with the addition of a national program of comparative effectiveness research, requires an increased supply of researchers who are skilled at working with public officials and are rewarded by their institutions and professional peers for doing so. Staff members of the EPCs from which DERP commissions systematic reviews are the only investigators who collaborate with public officials to plan as well as conduct such research on a regular basis. These researchers accept priorities for reviewing drug classes that are established by the public officials who govern DERP, collaborate with them to formulate key questions, interpret the findings of systematic reviews, and discuss appropriate responses to critical comments about drafts and published reviews.[25]

Few researchers have had training or experience that prepares them for the interactive work of convergence. Most of them, like their colleagues in other areas of social science and biomedicine, define their principal professional work as conducting research that they initiate in order to write articles, reports, systematic reviews, and sometimes books. Some of them occasionally advise policymakers or members of their staff on questions that they have previously investigated. Most of them have, however, been admonished by mentors and peers to regard advising, teaching, community and university service, and sometimes even clinical practice, as distractions from their more important work of generating and investigating hypotheses.

Most of the academic researchers who study health services have lower prestige and less financial support than their colleagues in the basic sciences and clinical disciplines. Many of them have struggled for promotion, tenure, and research funding. Because of their relatively low status, they are particularly sensitive about engaging in research that could be labeled as "contract" or "targeted"; that is, research for which funders set the questions. They perceive, correctly, that association with targeted research could lower their status among academic colleagues. Many of them have told intermediaries who ask them to collaborate with public officials that doing such research would misuse their time.

In a simplistic definition, targeted research is the essence of convergence. But working collaboratively with policymakers requires skills that are not commonly associated with targeted research. These skills include the ability to discuss with policymakers the most helpful key questions that can be answered with available evidence, to analyze data rigorously while working to strict deadlines, and to interpret and defend methodology and findings to diverse and frequently hostile audiences.

Many health services researchers do the work of convergence effectively. There are, however, more demands on their time than they can meet. Mark Helfand's contributions to DERP are described in Chapter 4. A partial list of others includes Nick Black, Iain Chalmers, and Mike Clarke (United Kingdom), Lisa Bero and Kay Dickersin (United States), Curt Furberg (Sweden and the United States), Jeremy Grimshaw (Scotland and Canada), Steven Leeder (Australia), Andrew Oxman (Norway, Canada and the United States), Peter Tugwell (United Kingdom and Canada), and Jimmy Volmink (South Africa).

These researchers and some of their colleagues are raising the prestige of the scientific work that convergence requires. Leeder has been a dean of both public health and medicine and now directs the Menzies Centre for Health Policy of the University of Sydney and the Australian National University. Tugwell chaired the Department of Medicine at the University of Ottawa and before that the Department of Clinical Epidemiology at McMaster University. He now directs the Centre for Global Health at the University of Ottawa. Queen Elizabeth II knighted Chalmers for his science and public service. Oxman has been both a professor (at McMaster) and a public official (in Norway). Volmink, who directed the South African Cochrane Centre of the Medical Research Council, became a department chairman at the University of Cape Town and is now deputy dean (research) in Stellenbosch University's Faculty of Health Sciences at Tygerberg, South Africa.

POLITICAL SUPPORT FOR CONVERGENCE

Evidence that convergence improves the quality of care and restrains the growth of its costs is necessary for its sustainability. But it is not sufficient.

Convergence can be sustained in the United States only if leaders of general government in many states continue to consider it to be both helpful and politically feasible and help to persuade members of Congress and federal officials to use the new program of comparative effectiveness research to enhance convergence in coverage under Medicare. Each of these leaders of state government regularly weighs evidence about support for and antagonism to the results of convergence from groups that speak for professions and provider organizations, business, health insurance plans, patients, and voters. They will also accord close attention to opinions about the benefits and political costs of convergence among their colleagues in government.

Growing appreciation among physicians of the usefulness of evidence-based health research contributes to the political legitimacy of convergence. Many of the members and staff of medical specialty societies who write and review clinical practice guidelines now accord more weight to the findings of systematic reviews than they do to individual studies. Major medical journals frequently publish systematic reviews and require that they meet high standards. The *Lancet*, for example, requires authors of papers based on RCTs to submit their protocols for review when they begin their research (in order to detect bias) and authors of systematic reviews to adhere to the standards of the Cochrane Collaboration. Teachers of clinical medicine increasingly expect undergraduate medical students, residents, and clinical fellows to be familiar with the best available evidence from research.[26]

A systematic review of "The Relationship between Clinical Experience and Quality of Care," published in 2005, documented growing attention to evidence-based health research among specialists in internal medicine. The authors found that "evidence-based medicine has been widely adopted and quality assurance techniques . . . are frequently used" among younger internists. In contrast, "physicians who have been in practice longer may be at risk for providing lower-quality care."[27]

Physicians who make clinical policy for integrated health systems and large hospital systems regularly use evidence-based health research to inform policy for drug formularies, processes to prevent harm to patients, and quality improvement. Notable examples of health and hospital systems that use this research include Ascension Health, Intermountain Healthcare, Kaiser Permanente, the Group Health Cooperative of Puget Sound, HealthPartners, and Sutter Health. David Pryor, chief medical officer of Ascension, said in 2008, for example, that his goal is to use the best evidence in creating "a high reliability culture" within that large national organization.[28] Similarly, medical directors of the largest health insurance plans—notably, Aetna, Anthem, and the Blue Cross and Blue Shield

Association on behalf of its members—use independent research, some of which they conduct internally.

There is also evidence of change in the division of authority within the medical profession that for decades inhibited the influence of research evaluating health services on clinical practice. Mandatory recertification is a powerful incentive for specialists to remain current with the literature on effectiveness and quality. State medical societies are increasingly comfortable with the appointment of academic physicians to state licensing boards, and even as their chairs and full-time executives. James Thompson, president of the Federation of State Medical Boards (FSMB) until 2008, is a former dean of medicine.

The FSMB and the National Board of Medical Examiners recently overcame vehement opposition from the AMA and state societies to requiring independent assessment of physicians' clinical skills as part of the Medical Licensing Examination. Over a ten-year period required assessment will prevent nine million encounters between patients and deficient physicians, Thompson estimates. Thompson has also been a leader in mobilizing major associations of physicians in an Alliance for Physician Competence, which in 2008 issued a document defining "good medical practice."[29]

A limitation on the sustainability of convergence is that most of it has occurred in state government. However, the physicians who are responsible for health benefits in a few very large companies seek the best available evidence and apply it in making decisions about coverage and the relative quality of provider organizations. Robert Galvin at General Electric and Clarion E. Johnson Jr. at ExxonMobil are notable examples. Galvin, for example, facilitated the writing and publication of a case study assessing value-based purchasing at General Electric.[30] Johnson required physicians on his staff to participate in a workshop on the methodology of systematic reviews offered by the U.S. Cochrane Center.

Several of the approximately one hundred local and regional organizations that pool employers' purchasing power in markets for health services also promote the convergence of research and policy. Examples include the Pacific Business Group on Health and the Mid-West Business Group on Health. The Wisconsin Collaborative for Healthcare Quality measures and reports publicly on behalf of a consortium of major employers. Chris Queram, its chief executive, formerly directed The Alliance, an employer purchasing group in that state.

Galvin, Peter Lee and David Lansky of the Pacific Business Group, and other proponents of the convergence of research, policy, and practice have helped to establish and sustain national organizations that focus employers' attention on the relationship among quality, safety and cost. These organizations include the Leapfrog Group, Bridges to Excellence, and the Consumer-Purchaser Disclosure Project.

These private sector initiatives have had limited success. Galvin and Suzanne Delbanco, then chief executive of Leapfrog, reported in 2005 that only a "small portion" of employers had used its "tools to drive value-based purchasing." They cited a study that found that "80% of large employers lacked confidence in their ability to address cost and quality in the health care system." Moreover, very few employers had staff with expertise in evaluating health services, and the consulting firms that many employers hired to do this work frequently "develop their own criteria rather than using standard approaches," which "increases confusion."[31]

Galvin and Delbanco described other impediments to employers pooling their considerable purchasing power despite evidence that low-quality care is ineffective and expensive. Senior managers, even in large companies, "shy away from" decisions to limit coverage and choice among providers that are "likely to be unpopular with employees." Mid-size and small firms can only afford to employ "human resources generalists." In the smallest firms, these generalists often rely on insurance brokers for advice. Moreover, many employers are "too closely aligned with providers through service on hospital boards, or selling them goods and services."[32]

Many business executives are, moreover, reluctant to learn from the experience of state government because they assume that markets are always more efficient than government. Two initiatives of the Employee Benefit Research Institute (EBRI), an organization that is supported mainly by the private sector and respected for its research, exemplify this ideological divide. Dallas Salisbury, the president of EBRI, arranged for Mark Gibson and Siri Childs, who represents the state of Washington on the DERP governance, to describe DERP and its results to the senior vice president for human resources of a global corporation and members of his staff. The senior vice president insisted that the corporation's negotiations with suppliers of prescriptions drugs, which were based on its purchasing power, yielded lower prices than DERP reviews applied through PDLs. Childs asked what the corporation paid for several expensive drugs. Then she displayed data from Washington documenting both lower prices and substantial shifts in market share for these drugs.

Similarly, the Milbank Memorial Fund and EBRI commissioned a report by Mark Gibson and John Santa, "Designing Benefits with Evidence in Mind," which was published in 2006. Gibson and Santa described what they had learned about using research findings to design coverage as a result of their work with the Oregon Health Plan and DERP. Paul Fronstin, the senior health economist at EBRI, said in 2008 that he had no "evidence that any EBRI members read it."[33]

Increasing attention to problems of quality and safety in health care by print and electronic media could, however, encourage convergence in the private sector. Galvin, for instance, was more optimistic about employer "inventiveness in U.S. health care reform" in 2008 than in earlier articles. Employers' "support for reform," he wrote, "will be contingent on policies that drive improvements in cost containment and quality of care."[34]

Quality and safety have been major news stories since the IOM report of 1999 that documented many unnecessary deaths in hospitals. For example, a finding by investigators at RAND in 2003 that only a small percentage of Americans receive appropriate care for leading chronic diseases received widespread coverage.[35] Favorable media accounts of the success of the "Hundred Thousand Lives Campaign" to improve safety in hospitals in 2005 assisted the Institute for Healthcare Improvement, its organizer, in raising its goal to saving five million lives between 2006 and 2008.

Major news outlets now regularly cover findings from new systematic reviews. By 2005, the *Wall Street Journal*, the Associated Press, and leading weekly news magazines were using the term without defining it; editors assumed that readers knew that these reviews used a persuasive methodology.

Media reporting on systematic reviews has significant external support. The Annenberg Foundation and the Carnegie Corporation of New York made grants in 2005 to establish a news service that sends stories about new systematic reviews to media outlets. The Gates Foundation subsequently made a grant to the news service's parent organization, the Center for the Advancement of Health (CAH), to write stories about reviews of particular interest to media in low- and middle-income countries. Jessie Gruman, president of the CAH, reports that the service distributes "stories on around 150 systematic reviews a year." CAH is now shifting its emphasis from systematic reviews of all health interventions to "looking for ones that are directly relevant to individuals engaging in their health and health care."[36]

A growing number of journalists understand the methods of systematic reviews and use them in stories. The National Association of Health Journalists (NAHJ) has held seminars about the methodology of systematic reviews at several of its annual meetings. These seminars have been lead by Ray Moynihan, an Australian reporter who has been covering convergence since the early 1990s.[37] Andrew Holtz, the executive director of NAHJ and a former medical reporter for CNN, serves on the Advisory Board of the U.S. Cochrane Center.

Some major outlets for information about medical research have, however, been unenthusiastic about systematic reviews. The *New England Journal of Medicine (NEJM)* rejected articles based on systematic reviews for many years, allegedly because its statistical consultant was critical of meta-analysis, a methodology for pooling data from RCTs that is a component of many reviews. In 2007, however, the *NEJM* published an article based on a meta-analysis that called attention to adverse events associated with Avandia, a drug for treating diabetes. A front-page article and then an editorial in the *New York Times*, however, made the misleading statement that a meta-analysis is inferior to a single well-designed randomized trial.[38]

The public is learning about the findings of systematic reviews from other sources. *Consumer Reports Best Buy Drugs®*, described in Chapter 4 because it is based on reviews commissioned by DERP, has been the subject of stories on the nightly news programs of ABC and CBS and been featured by Oprah Winfrey.[39] In 2006, Minnesota became the third of what by 2008 were six states to conduct a campaign promoting *Best Buy Drugs*. Consumers Union collaborated on the campaign with the state's governor, the Minnesota Medical Association and the state's Senior Federation. Launching the campaign, Minnesota Governor Tim Pawlenty told a reporter for the Associated Press, "We bought prescription medicines stupidly." A pharmacy expert at the University of Minnesota, Stephen Schondelmeyer, told the reporter, "The information [in *Best Buy Drugs*] could change the pharmaceutical marketplace within a few years if the site catches on with consumers." A spokesman for the Pharmaceutical Research and Manufacturers Association of America (PhRMA), agreed that "this is not a bad effort" and offered a subdued version of the industry's standard complaint against DERP: "but we have some questions about the methodology behind *Best Buy Drugs*."[40]

Gail Shearer of Consumers Union reports that *Best Buy Drugs* is reaching consumers in new ways. The Wisconsin Education Association Trust (WEAT), which manages pharmaceutical benefits for retired teachers, mailed a two-page summary of the DERP review of proton pump inhibitors to members who used these drugs. WEAT estimated that the mailing yielded about $450,000 in savings to consumers.[41] Medco Health Solutions, the nation's largest pharmacy benefit manager (PBM), subsequently mailed a summary of the DERP review of statins (a class of drugs to lower cholesterol) to about one million of its members. Medco estimated that the mailing saved consumers about $8 million. Shearer says that "our hope now is to figure out how to do this on a much larger scale."

The public has increasing access to the findings of systematic reviews on the Web. Abstracts of Cochrane reviews are available without charge. "More than half the world's consumers and health professionals" have free access to the entire Cochrane Library as a result of subscriptions by central government in Australia, Finland, India, Ireland, the countries of Latin America and the Caribbean, New Zealand, Norway, Poland, Sweden, and the United Kingdom. Three Canadian provinces and a territory offered free access until April 2009, when the Canadian Cochrane Network and Centre in partnership with the Canadian Health Libraries Association secured a national license under a pilot project. The Health Quality Council of Saskatchewan, a public body, subsidizes the training of librarians to help citizens interpret Cochrane reviews. More than four million individuals visited the Cochrane Library in 2007. A petition began to circulate in 2007 to expand access to Cochrane reviews to everyone in the European Union.[42] The National Library of Medicine has discussed a national site license with Wiley InterScience, publisher of the Cochrane Library. Meanwhile individual and institutional subscriptions to the Library in the United States continue to increase.

Wyoming is the only American jurisdiction that offers free access to the entire Cochrane Library. State Senator and Health Committee Chair Charles Scott, who is also a member of the RSG Steering Committee, obtained a subsidy for this subscription because he believes that good information creates and maintains free markets. Several years earlier, Scott had arranged Wyoming's membership in DERP for the same libertarian reason.

Peer-reviewed journals, including the Cochrane Library, unexpectedly contributed to making research findings more accessible to policymakers and the public over the past decade by requiring authors to submit structured abstracts of their articles. These abstracts summarize under separate headings the purpose, research questions, methodology, results, and conclusions of articles. Most journals make structured abstracts available without charge on the Web.

But abstracts, even when structured, can mislead readers. Articles by methodologists report that many abstracts contain erroneous data.[43] Moreover, most readers who access abstracts on the Web do not know whether the articles they summarize have received single- (the referee is anonymous) or double-blinded peer review or whether authors and referees have declared potential conflicts of interest.

Policymakers will assess increasing public interest in evidence-based health research among health professionals and the public in the context of contradictory information. Direct-to-consumer advertising by pharmaceutical companies (and, increasingly, by manufacturers of implantable devices) is a source of substantial income for print and electronic publications. Drug and device manufacturers continue to market heavily to physicians, despite negative publicity about their sales methods and court decisions against drug companies for marketing their products for purposes not approved by the Food and Drug Administration.

Some of these impediments to sustaining convergence could be offset by public and institutional policy. Policymakers who pioneered in convergence have helped to pass laws requiring physicians to disclose income and gifts from manufacturers of pharmaceutical drugs and, in some states, medical devices as well. Lee Greenfield, for example, carried a bill in the Minnesota legislature requiring physicians to disclose income from drug manufacturers in 1993 because, as he told the *New York Times* in 2007, "Why do we want [manufacturers] bribing doctors to use what may not be the best or most cost-effective drug for the patient . . .?"[44] Six states and the District of Columbia now have similar laws.[45] In 2008, the U.S. Senate considered a bill requiring manufacturers of drugs and medical devices to report gifts to physicians. Major manufacturers supported the bill after its sponsors agreed to raise the reporting minimum from $25 to $500 and to reduce the range of fines for each violation from $10,000–$100,000 to $1,000–$5,000.[46]

Moreover, leaders of influential organizations of physicians are advocating institutional policy to mitigate what a group of medical luminaries called in 2006 the "conflicts of interest that still characterize the relationship between physicians and the health care industry." This group, convened by the American Board of Internal Medicine Foundation and an academic center financed by George Soros's Open Society Institute, recommended that academic medical centers "take the lead in eliminating" such conflicts.[47] In 2008, a panel of academic physicians and pharmaceutical company executives convened by the Association of American Medical Colleges and the Association of American Universities recommended new institutional standards for avoiding conflicts of interest.[48]

The pharmaceutical industry, or segments of it, may be adapting to evidence of support for convergence. An Arkansas official told a reporter for the *Arkansas Democrat-Gazette* in 2006 that "we've actually gotten more compliments from manufacturers than complaints because of the fairness of the [PDL] system."[49] In 2007, Research and Markets, which calls itself the "world's largest market research resource," sought subscribers to a new report, *State Activities: Impact on the U.S. Pharmaceutical Industry*. In its marketing brochure, the firm noted the rapid expansion of state policymaking for prescription drugs, especially the spread of PDLs, and identified DERP's role. "Can pharmaceutical companies turn this situation around?" the firm's brochure asked. They can, it answered, only if manufacturers "adjust their marketing strategies to the requirements of increasingly vigilant" states and seek opportunities to "build mutually beneficial relationships" with them.[50]

States are also becoming more aggressive in using findings from independent research in making policy for prescription drugs. Six states have programs to counter "detailing" to physicians by sales representatives of the pharmaceutical industry with visitors who offer evidence from independent research. Seven other states are considering such programs. Physicians in the Canadian provinces of Alberta, British Columbia, Nova Scotia, and Saskatchewan can earn continuing medical education credit for meeting with such "academic detailers."[51] State officials are also sharing information about policy for prescription drugs and the industry's behavior through the newsletter and meetings of the National Legislative Association on Prescription Drug Prices (NLARx).

WHAT NEXT?

As a result of the events described in this book, evidence from independent research is informing the making of significant health policy in many American states. Findings from research are contributing to policy, just as competition for scarce public resources, the actions of interest and advocacy groups, public opinion, and the values of policymakers also contribute to it.

The politics of convergence could, for example, countervail against pressure on state legislators by advocates and organizations of health professionals to mandate coverage of health services. When legislators consider proposed mandates, they are overwhelmed by competing claims about findings from research that could be subject to rigorous review.[52] At least twenty-six states have created processes for reviewing proposed mandates since the early 1990s. A majority of these states, according to a recent review of enabling statutes, "specified a prospective review approach and only one law used an exclusively retrospective review."

Mandated benefit review is, however, still a weak example of convergence. There is a "substantial amount of variation with regards to the designated reviewers, time frames for conducting reviews, and criteria used in the review."[53] Investigators in one state said, for example, that they conduct systematic reviews: but one of their so-called systematic reviews included only one primary study.

Mandated benefit reviews have contributed to policy in some states. The Maryland legislature, for instance, has since 1998 required its Health Care Access and Cost Commission (now the Health Care Commission) to "annually assess the financial, social and medical impact of proposed mandates."[54] According to John Colmers, the founding executive director of the commission, and now Maryland secretary of health and mental hygiene, this requirement "tended to reduce, but not eliminate the appetite to enact further mandates."[55] Similarly, in the early 1990s, the Oregon Health Plan (OHP) replaced mandates of Medicaid services with legislative action on a budget for a list of services proposed by a commission. Mark Gibson, who was chief of staff to the state Senate president during the introduction of the OHP, recalls that Oregon legislators were pleased to "let the technical process" determine "what priority a given service had . . . and get out of playing referee among requestors."[56]

The processes through which convergence operates in each state usually take account of the limits of research and changes in methods and findings. Randomized controlled trials (RCTs) and systematic reviews have made the most important contributions to the success of convergence in coverage for prescription drugs. But these methodologies are not always the most appropriate ways to address other important questions to which policymakers want answers. They have, for example, limited application for evaluating the effectiveness of medical devices, surgical procedures, and changes in processes of care in order to improve its safety and quality.

There is considerable scope for expanding convergence that relies on rigorous evidence reviews that use a variety of methods. States are building on the success of PDLs and the work of DERP. At least fourteen states are using their PDLs for other programs than Medicaid, according to a 2008 report from the National Conference of State Legislatures.[57] A state official reported in 2008 that "we are driving toward using the PDL for public employees." Other states report that managed care plans and hospitals, as another official put it, "want to negotiate their [pharmaceutical] contracts to match ours."

Convergence appears to be most advanced in the state of Washington. The state requires that systematic reviews inform decisions about prescription drug coverage for public employees and persons who receive services under its workers' compensation program, as well as under Medicaid. Almost 800,000 people participated in these programs at the end of 2008. Under the leadership of Washington State Representative Eileen Cody, the chair of the Health Committee of the House and an oncology nurse practitioner, the state has also mandated the use of the best evidence to develop performance measures and financial incentives to improve quality among providers of mental health, chemical dependency, juvenile rehabilitation, and child welfare services. It has used evidence reviews to devise guidelines for treating pain. The legislature has funded a technology assessment program that commissions systematic reviews and permitted the health agency to finance reviews with savings from its PDL.[58]

A regulation adopted by the Medicaid agency in Kansas in 2001 establishes a hierarchy of evidence for responding to physicians' requests to authorize particular interventions as "medically necessary." The state requires that "scientific evidence [about] each existing intervention shall be considered first and, to the greatest extent possible shall be the basis for determinations of medical necessity." Scientific evidence for coverage must demonstrate that the "health intervention is known to be effective in improving health outcomes." In the absence of such evidence, decisions are based on "professional standards of care," and in the absence of such standards, on "expert opinion."[59]

The history of this regulation encapsulates the brief history of the convergence of research and governance policymaking for health in American states. Nialson Lee, then the administrator of healthcare systems and policy for Kansas Medicaid, attended a workshop sponsored by the User Liaison Program in 2000. He recalled in 2008 that "there was a section discussing the importance of a good medical necessity statement." Lee and the Medical Workgroup of his agency subsequently reviewed medical necessity policies from other states and private groups. They found that a report commissioned from the Stanford University Center for Health Policy by the California Healthcare Foundation (CHCF) was "perfect," Lee recalled. The Workgroup then "formatted [it] to Kansas regulations language" and implemented it.[60]

The Kansas regulation mandated the convergence of research and policy by establishing a hierarchy of evidence as the standard for decisions. The regulation described the relative validity and reliability of different types of evidence. The report for the CHCF, in contrast, focused on reducing variation in medical necessity decisions among the managed care plans that served Medicaid recipients. It mentioned standards of evidence vaguely and did not specify a hierarchy. An intervention must merely be "known to be effective" in order to be judged medically necessary, the authors wrote. One of them recalled in 2008, however, that David Eddy, a noted researcher on health services who facilitated the workshop that preceded the report, had "made it clear to the participants that the hierarchy of evidence was meant to be followed in decision-making."[61]

The Kansas regulation is a significant contribution to establishing the principle that the most effective convergence requires attention to the best available independent evidence. The state of Washington has, less explicitly, also established evidentiary standards for medical necessity. No other state appears to have adopted similar regulations.

Medical necessity remains a sensitive political issue in both the public and private sectors. This sensitivity could explain why the Stanford Center's report did not include Eddy's advice about a hierarchy of evidence. Adjudicating physicians' insistence that the interventions they propose are medically necessary requires officials to weigh scientific evidence, professional judgment and, either explicitly or implicitly, considerations of cost. Setting explicit standards for medical necessity and putting the burden of proof on physicians and other providers may, at present, be beyond what the politics of convergence can achieve.

I began this book by describing immediate and underlying causes of the convergence of research findings and the process of policymaking for covering prescription drugs in state Medicaid programs. Then I presented a history of health services research in the United States, emphasizing how the politics of the health sector have influenced what researchers studied and the methods they used. Next I described how officials of state government became increasingly influential in health affairs and effective in making policy. I told the story of the Drug Effectiveness Review Project in Chapter 4 in order to exemplify how the competence of state officials and their understanding of the methods and uses of research evaluating health services made convergence possible and then made it successful. Finally, I assessed the politics of convergence in order to explain why it succeeded and to describe uncertainties about its future.

Convergence has been defended successfully in most of the states and is expanding in scope in many of them. A new arena of convergence for states could be "conditional coverage with evidence-development" in Medicaid, the State Children's Health Insurance Program, and coverage for current and retired state employees that draws on the experience of

Medicare regulators in the United States and similar programs in France, the United Kingdom, and the province of Ontario.[62]

Could the partial success of convergence in policy for health services be a model for using findings from independent research in other areas of policy? Systematic reviews commissioned by the Centers for Disease Control and Prevention (CDC) through its Task Force on Community Preventive Services have helped policymakers justify policy to ban smoking in public places and to end referrals of some adolescents from juvenile to adult courts and prisons. Many of the twenty-seven states that had established reporting systems for adverse events in hospitals and clinics by 2007 "demonstrate[ed] a growing intent to use [these systems] to promote quality improvement" by requiring research (called root-cause analysis) on these events. But no state has established a formal, transparent process under which independent systematic reviews and other research can inform policy for public health or patient safety.[63]

Convergence that is analogous to what is occurring in health policy could occur in other areas of policy, but it would have different political characteristics. The brief history of the federal Data Quality Act of 2000 demonstrates the difficulty of making and enforcing standards of evidence across policy areas. The act directed the Office of Management and Budget to issue governmentwide guidelines that "provide policy and procedural guidance to Federal agencies for ensuring and maximizing the quality, objectivity, utility, and integrity of information (including statistical information) disseminated by Federal agencies." However, journalists and many outraged scientists have complained that the guidelines have permitted corporations and their supporters to suppress information that threatens their interests.[64] Similarly, the Union of Concerned Scientists published an "A to Z Guide to Political Interference in Science" on its Web site, noting, "In recent years, scientists who work for and advise the federal government have seen their work manipulated, suppressed, distorted, while agencies have systematically limited . . . access to critical scientific information."[65] The appointment of distinguished scientists to policymaking positions at the beginning of the Obama administration has, however, stimulated new optimism about potential convergence.

The culture of health services may be more conducive to convergence than that of some other areas of policy. Biomedical science has earned profound respect among health professionals, policymakers, the press and the public for more than a century. As a result, health policy based on the best available evidence may sometimes restrain—though it never eliminates—efforts by commercial interests and advocates to promote coverage and prescribing that are based on research that lacks rigor or that is spun.

Interest and advocacy groups and many physicians continue to press to weaken or to narrow the scope of convergence in health policy. Australia, which was the first country to establish a formal process for using independent research to evaluate prescription drugs, has also been the first to experience new strategies by the pharmaceutical industry to weaken convergence.

A recent strategy of lobbyists for international drug companies in Australia has been to claim that according preference in coverage to the most effective drugs inhibits innovation in pharmaceutical research and is, therefore, detrimental to the Australian economy. Although researchers report that evidence of such inhibition is "ambivalent or contrary," the Labor Party government that took office in 2007, like its more conservative Liberal predecessor, has been sympathetic to the companies' argument.[66] Australian physicians, similarly, have recently succeeded in retaining government subsidy for prescribing anti-depressants to children despite the "federal Government's own drugs watchdog recommending that they not be taken by anyone under the age of 24."[67]

As this book went into production, a close student of policy for pharmaceutical drugs posted evidence on his blog that the industry had again used Australia as a laboratory for political tactics it would introduce in the United States. He reported that Pfizer's chairman and CEO Jeffrey Kindler and Stanford University Emeritus Professor of Law John Barton had informed Senator Max Baucus (D-Mont.), chairman of the U.S. Senate Committee on Finance, that they were convening "major stakeholders" to discuss ways "to ensure that pricing and reimbursement policies recognize and reward innovation" and "to set disciplines on government practices that undermine incentives for innovation."[68]

The antagonists of convergence will continue to exploit its fragility. I hope its friends continue to be effective in the politics and policymaking required to sustain and extend it.

Notes

PREFACE

1. Daniel M. Fox, "History and Health Policy: An Autobiographical Note on the Decline of Historicism," *Journal of Social History* 18, no. 3 (March 1985): 349–64.

2. Daniel M. Fox, *Power and Illness: The Failure and Future of American Health Policy* (Berkeley: University of California Press, 1993).

CHAPTER 1

1. In this chapter I cite factual statements and quotations for which there is a public record. I also identify a sample of sources for statements that will be documented more extensively in subsequent chapters. I do this in order to demonstrate that this book is based on research as well as on personal experience. I describe my sources and methods in the concluding section of this chapter. Thus the first citation is to a compilation of data: Richard Cauchi, *Pharmaceutical Preferred Drug Lists (PDLs)—State Medicaid and Beyond*, preliminary ed. (Denver, CO: National Conference of State Legislatures, rev. January 3, 2008); courtesy Richard Cauchi.

2. See, e.g., Henry J. Kaiser Family Foundation, "United States: Medicaid Enrollment as a Percent of Total Population, 2006" (most recent available), www.statehealthfacts.org/profileind.jsp?ind=199&cat=4&rgn=1 (accessed April 4, 2009).

3. William J. Novak, *The People's Welfare: Law and Regulation in Nineteenth-Century America* (Chapel Hill, NC: University of North Carolina Press, 1996), pp. 8, 252n20.

4. For the last two sentences: Robert Pear, "U.S. Appeals Court Backs State Efforts at Drug Cost Control," *New York Times*, April 6, 2004, www.nytimes.com/2004/04/06/politics/06DRUG.html (accessed April 4, 2009), is a reliable summary of these events.

5. Panos Kanavos and Uwe Reinhardt, "Reference Pricing for Drugs: Is It Compatible with U.S. Health Care?" *Health Affairs* 22, no. 3 (2003): 16–30, is an early (and perhaps the first) article on reference drug pricing in a major U.S. health policy journal. See also Steven G. Morgan et al., "Centralized Drug Review Processes in Australia, Canada, New Zealand and the United Kingdom," *Health Affairs* 25, no. 2 (2006): 337–47, for an overview of processes for reviewing drugs in other countries.

6. Ron Winslow, Laurie McGinley and Chris Adams, "Drug Prices—Why They Keep Soaring—Healing the System: States, Insurers Find Prescriptions for High Drug Costs—Michigan's Blue Cross Pushes Generics, While Vermont's Strong-Arms Producers—PhRMA Fights Back in Court," *Wall Street Journal*, September 11, 2002, A1.

7. *Informing Judgment: Case Studies of Health Policy and Research in Six Countries*, ed. Daniel M. Fox and Andrew D. Oxman (New York: Milbank Memorial Fund, 2001), www.milbank.org/reports/2001cochrane/010903cochrane.html (accessed April 4, 2009).

8. Archie Cochrane had proposed a program to evaluate interventions to improve health in a series of lectures sponsored by the Nuffield Trust in London in 1971, which were subsequently published as A. L. Cochrane, *Effectiveness and Efficiency: Random Reflections on Health Services* (London: Nuffield Provincial Hospitals Trust, 1972). For an introduction to the methods and uses of randomized controlled trials and systematic reviews, see Imogen Evans, Hazel Thornton, and Iain Chalmers, *Testing Treatments: Better Research for Better Health Care* (London: British Library, 2006); available at www.jameslindlibrary.org/testing-treatments.html (accessed April 4, 2009).

9. Iain Chalmers, Murray Enkin, and Mark Keirse, *Effective Care in Pregnancy and Childbirth*, 2 vols. (Oxford: Oxford University Press, 1989).

10. Earl Ubell, "Are Births as Safe as They Could Be?" *Parade*, February 7, 1993, p. 1.

11. For the history of this theory and its application to policy, see Daniel M. Fox, *Health Policies, Health Politics: The British and American Experience, 1911–1965* (Princeton, NJ: Princeton University Press, 1986).

12. A quarter of Americans lived in the suburbs in 1950, and a third in 1960; by 1970 suburbanites were a "solid majority" (*The New Suburban History*, ed. Kevin M. Krause and Thomas J. Sugrue [Chicago: University of Chicago Press, 2006], p. 1). Suburbanization contributed to the loss of the power of central cities in state government by accelerating the decline of political parties and the rise of interest-based politics, as described by Margaret Weir, "Central Cities' Loss of Power in State Politics," *Cityscape: A Journal of Policy Development and Research* 2, no. 2 (May 1996): 23–40. However, for a generally critical history of suburbanization, emphasizing the "loss of community in Metropolitan America," see Kenneth T. Jackson, *Crabgrass Frontier: The Suburbanization of the United States* (New York: Oxford University Press, 1985). Jackson does acknowledge that families that moved

to suburbs "were looking for good schools, private space and personal safety" (p. 244).

13. Congressional Budget Office, "Technological Change and the Growth of Health Care Spending," January 2008, www.cbo.gov/doc.cfm?index=8947 (accessed April 4, 2009).

14. For these issues, see *Medical Care Output and Productivity*, ed. David M. Cutler and Ernst R. Berndt, NBER Studies in Income and Wealth, vol. 62 (Chicago: University of Chicago Press, 2001), and David M. Cutler, *Your Money or Your Life: Strong Medicine for America's Health Care System* (New York: Oxford University Press, 2005).

15. This section is based on Daniel M. Fox, *Power and Illness: The Failure and Future of American Health Policy* (Berkeley: University of California Press, 1993).

16. Lewis Thomas, "The Technology of Medicine," in id., *The Lives of a Cell* (New York: Viking Press, 1974).

17. Daniel M. Fox and Daniel C. Schaffer, "Tax Policy as Social Policy: Cafeteria Plans, 1978–1985," *Journal of Health Politics, Policy and Law* 12 (Winter 1987): 609–64.

CHAPTER 2

1. Thomas Neville Bonner, *Iconoclast: Abraham Flexner and a Life in Learning* (Baltimore: Johns Hopkins University Press, 2002).

2. Stephen J. Kunitz, *The Health of Populations: General Theories and Particular Realities* (New York: Oxford University Press, 2007), pp. 16–26, is an insightful account of the science and politics of these diseases and cites other relevant literature.

3. Daniel M. Fox, *Health Policies, Health Politics: The British and American Experience, 1911–1965* (Princeton, NJ: Princeton University Press, 1986), pp. 38–42, and "Abraham Flexner's Unpublished Report: Foundations and Medical Education, 1909–1928, *Bulletin of the History of Medicine* 54 (Winter 1980): 475–96. On Davis, see also Jonathan Engel, *Doctors and Reformers: Discussion and Debate over Health Policy, 1925–1950* (Columbia, SC: University of South Carolina Press, 2002), pp. 17–19.

4. Engel, *Doctors and Reformers*, pp. 11–52, is the best overview of the history of CCMC.

5. Fox, *Health Policies, Health Politics*, n. 3 above, pp. 45–51, is a controversial analysis of the reformers' political miscalculation and their use of research to amplify it. Jennifer Klein, *For All These Rights: Business, Labor, and the Shaping of America's Public-Private Welfare State* (Princeton, NJ: Princeton University Press, 2003), pp. 119–21, provides additional evidence of how the reformers blurred the distinction between research and advocacy.

6. See Daniel M. Fox, "The Significance of the Milbank Memorial Fund for Policy: An Assessment at Its Centennial," *Milbank Quarterly* 84, no. 1

(2006): 1–32, for primary sources for the story in this and in subsequent paragraphs on the Fund.

7. Fox, *Health Policies, Health Politics*, n. 3 above, pp. 91–93.

8. See Daniel M. Fox, *Economists and Health Care* (New York: Prodist, 1979), 23–24, for sources that indicate that the successful censorship of Friedman was well known among economists. Lanny Ebenstein, *Milton Friedman: A Biography* (New York: Palgrave Macmillan, 2007) adds additional details.

9. Fox, *Economists*, n. 8 above, pp. 23, 26, 87 (the latter within a memoir by Herbert Klarman).

10. Daniel M. Fox, *Power and Illness: The Failure and Future of American Health Policy* (Berkeley: University of California Press, 1993), pp. 34–36.

11. George St. J. Perrott and Dorothy F. Holland, "Population Trends and Problems of Public Health," *Milbank Memorial Fund Quarterly* 18, no. 4 (1940): 359–92; reprinted in *Milbank Quarterly* 83, no. 4 (2005): 569–608.

12. Fox, *Health Policies, Health Politics*, n. 3 above, pp. 115–23.

13. Emily K. Abel, Elizabeth Fee, and T. M. Brown, "Milton I. Roemer: Advocate of Social Medicine, International Health, and National Health Insurance," *American Journal of Public Health* 98, no. 9 (September 2008): 3–5.

14. Harry M. Marks, *The Progress of Experiment: Science and Therapeutic Reform in the United States, 1900–1990* (Cambridge: Cambridge University Press, 1997), pp. 42–70; Fox, *Power and Illness*, n. 10 above, pp. 42–44.

15. Fox, *Power and Illness*, 44–47. Two statements by principals in the new research center exemplify my generalizations. In a lecture, "The Value of Research in Chronic Care," given at a conference convened in 1936 to celebrate the opening of the research center on Welfare Island, Alfred Cohn said, "The methods of natural science are regarded as appropriate for use in the clinic" (Alfred Cohn Papers, Rockefeller Archives Center, Tarrytown, NY, Box 21v, F21). Similarly, David Seegal, a prominent investigator at the center wrote in 1938 that "increased investigation in the basic sciences is imperative if chronic diseases are to be better controlled" ("The Problem of Chronic Disease: Investigation of Chronic Diseases under Municipal Sponsorship in the Department of Hospitals of New York City," *Hospitals* 12 [March 1938]: 33–39).

16. For the "first cooperative controlled trial," see Scott H. Podolsky, *Pneumonia before Antibiotics: Therapeutic Evolution and Evaluation in Twentieth-Century America* (Baltimore: Johns Hopkins University Press, 2006), p. 5. I draw the other evidence in this paragraph from archival sources listed on pp. 146–47 of *Power and Illness*, n. 10 above. To my embarrassment I discovered while writing this book that the precise citations to sources in that book relevant to this paragraph disappeared during its production, with a gap in numbering; neither I nor the copy editor nor any reviewer noticed that

several pages of citations are missing. I hope to compensate for this error in a subsequent article.

17. Klein, *For All These Rights*, n. 5 above, p. 120.

18. Susan Reverby, "Stealing the Golden Eggs: Ernest Amory Codman and the Science of Management in Medicine, *Bulletin of the History of Medicine* 55, no. 1 (1981): 156–71. Avedis Donabedian, "The End Results of Health Care: Ernest Codman's Contribution to Quality Assessment and Beyond," *Milbank Quarterly* 67, no. 2 (1989): 233–56; Donald M. Berwick, "E. A. Codman and the Rhetoric of Battle: A Commentary," ibid.: 262–67.

19. Jeanne Daly, *Evidence-Based Medicine and the Search for a Science of Clinical Care* (Berkeley: University of California Press and the Milbank Memorial Fund, 2005), pp. 15, 52; Paul made his proposal in his presidential address to the American Society of Clinical Investigation. Howell writes that his colleagues in the ASCI were unmoved because "compared with the traditional sciences health services and outcomes research could be seen as less scholarly and more ideological." J. Howell, "A History of the American Society for Clinical Investigation," *Journal of Clinical Investigation* 119, no. 4 (April 2009): 693.

20. Fox, *Health Policies, Health Politics*, n. 3 above, p. 87.

21. Benjamin Toth, "Clinical Trials in British Medicine 1858–1948, with Special Reference to the Development of the Randomised Controlled Trial" (PhD diss., University of Bristol, 1998), p. 198, www.jameslindlibrary.org/pdf/theses/toth-1998.pdf (accessed April 11, 2009).

22. David E. Lilienfeld, "Celebration: William Farr (1807–1883)—An Appreciation on the 200th Anniversary of His Birth," *International Journal of Epidemiology* 36, no. 5 (2007): 985–87; John Eyler, *Victorian Social Medicine: The Ideas and Methods of William Farr* (Baltimore: Johns Hopkins University Press, 1979).

23. Dorothy Porter, "How Did Social Medicine Evolve, and Where Is It Heading?" *PLoS Medicine* 3, no. 10 (October 24, 2006), www.plosmedicine.org/article/info:doi/10.1371/journal.pmed.0030399 (accessed April 5, 2009).

24. Daniel M. Fox, "The National Health Service and the Second World War: The Elaboration of Consensus," in *War and Social Change: British Society in the Second World War*, ed. Harold L. Smith (Manchester, UK: Manchester University Press, 1986), pp. 32–57; Fox, *Health Policies, Health Politics*, n. 3 above, pp. 94–114.

25. Ann Oakley, *Man and Wife: Richard and Kay Titmuss: My Parents' Early Years* (London: HarperCollins, 1996).

26. Daniel M. Fox, "Politics Matter: Re-Reading Abel Smith's History of Hospitals," *Journal of Health Services Research and Policy* 10, no. 3 (July 2005): 187–88.

27. A. L. Cochrane, with Max Blythe, *One Man's Medicine: An Autobiography of Professor Archie Cochrane* (London: BMJ Books, 1989), 45; Iain Chalmers, "Archie Cochrane (1909–1988)," www.jameslindlibrary.org/

trial_records/20th_Century/1940s/cochrane/cochrane_biog.html   (accessed April 11 2009).

28. Michael Marmot, "Early Pioneers of Epidemiology," review of *The Development of Modern Epidemiology: Personal Reports from Those Who Were There,* ed. Walter W. Holland, Jørn Olsen, and Charles du V. Florey (Oxford: Oxford University Press, 2007), *Lancet* 370 (December 1, 2007): 1819–20; see also *Making Health Policy: Networks in Research and Policy after 1945,* ed. Virginia Berridge, Wellcome Series in the History of Medicine, *Clio Medica* 75 (New York: Rodopi, 2005). Another useful essay, that supports the interpretation in this section is Nick Black, "Health Services Research: The Gradual Encroachment of Ideas" (unpublished MS, London School of Hygiene and Tropical Medicine, December 2008). In the Preface to this book I explain why, for most of my career, I wrote in two distinct voices, those of the Bureaucrat and the Narrator. If I had, like my predecessors (and many of my contemporaries) in Britain, devised another voice, the Advocate, I would have compromised my career as a researcher and been of no use to policymakers.

29. Fox, "Significance of the Milbank Memorial Fund," n. 6 above.

30. Fox, *Power and Illness,* n. 10 above, pp. 30–55; Lester Breslow, "Measuring Health in Its Third Era: (unpublished MS, 2008), pp. 10, 13; see also Alan M. Brandt and Martha Gardner, "Antagonism and Accommodation: Interpreting the Relationship between Public Health and Medicine in the United States during the 20th Century," *American Journal of Public Health* 90, no. 5 (May 2000): 707–15.

31. Marks, *Progress of Experiment,* n. 14 above, pp. 60–70; Podolsky, *Pneumonia before Antibiotics,* n. 16 above, passim.

32. Joyce Antler and Daniel M. Fox, "The Movement Toward a Safe Maternity: Physician Accountability in New York City, 1915–1940," *Bulletin of the History of Medicine* 50 (1976): 569–95.

33. Marks, *Progress of Experiment,* n. 14 above, pp. 113–28.

34. Toth, "Clinical Trials in British Medicine," n. 21, above, pp. 199–252. For an interpretation of the relationship between research and policy in the United Kingdom (and other countries) and the United States, see Harold L. Wilensky, "Social Science and the Public Agenda: Reflections on the Relation of Knowledge to Policy in the United States and Abroad," *Journal of Health Politics, Policy and Law* 22, no. 5 (October 1977): 1241–65.

35. Fox, *Power and Illness,* n. 10 above, pp. 52–55.

36. Fox, *Economists and Health Care,* n. 8 above, describes the history of postwar demand for research on health services, pp. 24–32. I contrast the immediate postwar years with the 1980s in Daniel M. Fox, "Health Policy and the Politics of Research in the United States, *Journal of Health Politics, Policy and Law* 15, no. 3 (Fall 1990): 481–99. For a sound history of research on health services that focuses on consensus, rather than, as I do, on conflict, see Odin W. Anderson, "Influence of Social and Economic Research on Public Policy in the Health Field: A Review," *Milbank Memorial Fund Quarterly* 44, no. 3, pt. 2 (July 1966): 11–51. See also Odin Anderson, *The Evolution of*

Health Services Research: Personal Reflections on Applied Social Science (San Francisco: Jossey-Bass, 1991). Kerr White, whose focus is on medicine and public health disciplines, accords less attention to the social sciences and offers a very different interpretation of the history of health services research than either Anderson or I do. Moreover, he focuses mainly on research funded by the federal government and accords high priority to describing his personal contribution to the early history of the field: Thomas McCarthy and Kerr L. White, "Origins of Health Services Research," *Health Services Research* 35, no. 2 (June 2000): 375–87; and in an oral history interview with Edward L. Berkowitz for the National Library of Medicine, History of Medicine Division in 1998, www.nlm.nih.gov/hmd/nichsr/white.html (accessed April 11, 2009).

37. Samuel W. Bloom, *The Word as Scalpel: A History of Medical Sociology* (New York: Oxford University Press, 2002); esp. chap. 9, "Becoming a Profession: The Role of the Private Foundations," pp. 181–213. On Milbank and deinstitutionalization, see Fox, "Significance of the Milbank Memorial Fund," n. 6 above. For foundations and health affairs more generally, see Daniel M. Fox, "Foundations and Health: Innovation, Marginalisation, and Relevance since 1900," in *The Roles and Contributions of Foundations*, ed. Helmut K. Anheier and David C. Hammack (Washington, DC: Brookings Institution Press, forthcoming).

38. Ivana Krajcinovic, *From Company Doctors to Managed Care: The United Mine Workers' Noble Experiment* (Ithaca, NY: ILR Press, an imprint of Cornell University Press, 1997), pp. 31, 55, 71, 133.

39. Fox, *Economists and Health Care*, n. 8 above, p. 29.

40. Bloom, *Word as Scalpel*, n. 37 above, p. 124. Odin Anderson was an exception. He conducted a study for the Health Information Foundation in 1959 that documented physicians' decisions leading to unnecessary hospital admissions in Massachusetts; see Anderson, *Evolution of Health Services Research*, n. 36 above.

41. Fox, *Economists and Health Care*, n. 8 above, p. 25.

42. Fox, *Health Policies, Health Politics*, n. 3 above, 207–12; a generally reliable account of the postwar history of AHCs is Irving J. Lewis and Cecil G. Sheps, *The Sick Citadel: The American Academic Medical Center and the Public Interest* (Cambridge, MA: Ballinger, 1983); Kenneth M. Ludmerer, *Time to Heal: American Medical Education from the Turn of the Century to the Era of Managed Care* (New York: Oxford University Press, 1999) is a thorough history, though it is focused more on medical education than on the role of AHCs in health policy.

43. Fox, *Economists and Health Care*, n. 8 above, p. 33; see also Edward Berkowitz's oral history interview with Herbert Klarman, www.nlm.gov/hmd/nichsr/klarman.html (accessed April 11, 2009).

44. Daniel M. Fox, "Sharing Governmental Authority: Blue Cross and Hospital Planning in New York City," *Journal of Health Politics, Policy and Law* 16, no. 4 (Winter 1991): 719–46.

45. I thank Kenneth L. Ludmerer and James Thompson for e-mail and conversation that improved my description of divided authority within medicine.

46. George Weisz, *Divide and Conquer: A Comparative History of Medical Specialization* (New York: Oxford University Press, 2006), p. 146.

47. Avedis Donabedian, "Evaluating the Quality of Medical Care," *Milbank Memorial Fund Quarterly* 44, no. 3, pt. 2 (1966): 166–203; reprinted in *Milbank Quarterly* 83, no. 4 (2005): 691–729.

48. Mindel C. Sheps, "Approaches to the Quality of Hospital Care," *Public Health Reports* 70 (1955): 877–86.

49. John Wennberg and Alan Gittlesohn, "Small Area Variation in Health Care Delivery: A Population-Based Health Information System Can Guide Planning and Regulatory Decision-Making," *Science* 182, no. 4117 (December 14, 1973): 1102–8.

50. Daniel M. Fox, "The Development of Priorities for Health Services Research: The National Center, 1974–1976," *Milbank Memorial Fund Quarterly* 54, no. 2 (Summer 1976): 237–48.

51. Richard M. Magraw, Daniel M. Fox, and Jerry L. Weston, "Health Professions Education and Public Policy: A Research Agenda," *Journal of Medical Education* 53, no. 7 (July 1978): 539–46.

52. John E. Wennberg, "Dealing with Medical Practice Variations: A Proposal for Action," *Health Affairs* 3, no. 2 (Summer 1984): 6–32. More recently, Wennberg and his colleagues have embraced research on effectiveness and policy to enhance physician accountability as tools to reduce unwarranted variation: see, e.g., John E. Wennberg, Shannon Brownlee, Elliott S. Fisher, Jonathan S. Skinner, and James N. Weinstein, *Improving Quality and Curbing Health Spending: Opportunities for the Obama Administration*, Dartmouth Atlas White Paper (Hanover, NH: Dartmouth Institute for Health Policy and Clinical Practice, 2008)

53. Marks, *Progress of Experiment*, n. 14 above, p. 133. The most complete study of RCTs in the United States in the 1970s and 1980s is still U.S. Congress, Office of Technology Assessment, *The Impact of Randomized Clinical Trials on Health Policy and Medical Practice*, OTA-BP-H-22 (Washington, DC: Office of Technology Assessment. 1983), http://govinfo .library.unt.edu/ota/Ota_4/DATA/1983/8310.PDF (accessed April 16, 2009).

54. American trialists were, however, reluctant to say that they were using methods that had evolved in Europe, as I discovered in the late 1980s as a member of an NIH committee that reviewed applications for community-based (in contrast to academic) trials of drugs to treat AIDS/HIV. In an invited letter to the editor, "It's Time to Open Clinical Drug Trials," *Brookings Review*, May 1991, p. 4, I summarized British criticism of American trials "as expensive and leading to inferior results" because of the narrow criteria used to recruit subjects.

55. Daly, *Evidence-Based Medicine*, n. 19 above, describes this work on the basis of interviews with most of these investigators. There is,

unfortunately, no similar secondary source for the mainstream observational researchers.

56. Sherry R. Arnstein and Alexander N. Christakis, *Perspectives on Technology Assessment* (Jerusalem, Israel: Science and Technology Publishers, 1975).

57. For an overview of the history of technology assessment, see Clifford S. Goodman, "HTA 101: Introduction to Health Technology Assessment," U.S. National Library of Medicine, National Information Center on Health Services Research and Health Care Technology, January 2004, updated 2007, www.nlm.nih.gov/nichsr/hta101/ta101_c1.html (accessed April 11, 2009). See also Richard A. Rettig, Peter D. Jacobson, Cynthia M. Farquhar, Wade M. Aubrey, *False Hope: Bone Marrow Transplantation for Breast Cancer* (New York: Oxford University Press, 2007), pp. 181–82. The *International Journal of Technology Assessment in Health Care* began publication in 1985. Its founding editor was an American and it was published by the New York office of Cambridge University Press. Nevertheless, a perverse effect of the history of TA in the United States has been that most of the best work in the field in this country could not be published in this journal because of the subscription business model that resulted from health politics.

58. U.S. Congress, Office of Technology Assessment, *Health Care Technology and Its Assessment in Eight Countries* (Washington, DC: OTA, 1995) remains the best source for the comparative history of TA. A meeting of British and American TA experts on TA convened by the Milbank Memorial Fund in 1999 to discuss cross-national collaboration failed because the British could not overcome their moral distaste for proprietary research and the Americans saw no prospect of TA becoming broadly available through publication in journals.

59. William L. Roper, William Winkenwerder, Glenn H. Hackbarth, and Henry Frakauer, "Effectiveness in Health Care: An Initiative to Evaluate and Improve Medical Practice," *New England Journal of Medicine* 319, no. 8 (November 3, 1988): 1197–1202. Another influential paper the same year was David M. Eddy and John Billings, "The Quality of Medical Evidence: Implications for Quality of Care," *Health Affairs* 7, no. 1 (January–February 1988): 19–32.

60. Bradford H. Gray, "The Legislative Battle over Health Services Research," *Health Affairs* 11, no. 4 (November-December, 1992): 38–56.

61. Bradford H. Gray, Michael K. Gusmano, and Sara Collins, "AHCPR and the Changing Politics of Health Services Research," http://content.healthaffairs.org/cgi/content/full/hlthaff.w3.283v1/DC1 (accessed April 11, 2009).

62. *To Err Is Human: Building a Safer Health System*, ed. Linda T. Kohn, Janet M. Corrigan, and Molla S. Donaldson (Washington, DC: National Academies Press, 2000); Committee on Quality of Health Care in America, *Crossing the Quality Chasm: A New Health System for the 21st Century* (Washington, DC: National Academies Press, 2001).

63. Nancy S. Sung et al. [eighteen co-authors], "Central Challenges Facing the National Clinical Research Enterprise," *JAMA* 289, no. 10 (March 12, 2003): 1278–87. This article had been cited in sixty other publications by 2008.

64. Reforming States Group, "State Initiatives on Prescription Drugs: Creating a More Functional Market," *Health Affairs* 22, no. 4 (July–August 2003): 128–36.

CHAPTER 3

1. There is a vast literature debating and dating labels characterizing the history of federalism. Recent publications that also call attention to the work of previous scholars include: Joseph F. Zimmerman, "National-State Relations: Cooperative Federalism in the 20th Century," *Publius* 31, no. 2 (Spring 2001): 15–30; Paul Posner, "The Politics of Coercive Federalism in the Bush Era," *Publius* 37, no. 3 (Summer 2007): 290–412; and Kimberley S. Johnson, *Congress and the New Federalism, 1877–1929* (Princeton, NJ: Princeton University Press, 2007).

2. Political scientists have told me repeatedly that this distinction between general and specialized government has no basis in the literature of their discipline, and that it is less useful than the descriptive models with which they are familiar. Most officials of general government who have heard me use the distinction say, on the other hand, that it is an apt characterization of their experience. I recently sought to explain this disagreement between persons who study politics and those who practice it. I found helpful the discussion of the problem of "political control" (in my terms, the relationship between generalists and specialists) in Kenneth J. Meier and Laurence J. O'Toole Jr., *Bureaucracy in a Democratic State: A Governance Perspective* (Baltimore: Johns Hopkins University Press, 2006), esp. pp. 21–44. Meier and O'Toole say that a major purpose of their book is to synthesize theories devised by the disciplines of political science and public administration. My description of generalists and specialists may fall into the gap they identify between these disciplines. Another useful analysis for understanding why the distinction between generalists and specialists distresses political scientists is in Daniel P. Carpenter, *The Forging of Bureaucratic Autonomy: Reputations, Networks and Policy Innovation in Executive Agencies, 1862–1928* (Princeton, NJ: Princeton University Press, 2001). Carpenter's definition of bureaucratic autonomy is consistent with part of my definition of specialized government ("when bureaucrats take actions consistent with their own wishes, actions to which politicians and organized interests defer" [p. 4]). In my formulation, however, the relationship between generalists and specialists is more frequently characterized by tension, and negotiations about such tension, than by deference.

3. This section is a revision and update of Daniel M. Fox, "The Competence of States and the Health of the Public," in *Health Policy Reform in America:*

Innovations from the States, ed. Howard M. Leichter, 2nd ed. (Armonk, NY: M. E. Sharpe, 1997), 29–46.

4. Brandeis's dissenting opinion in *New State Ice Co. v. Liebmann*, 285 US 262 (1932).

5. Martha Derthick, "Crossing Thresholds: Federalism in the 1960s," *Journal of Policy History* 8, no. 1 (1996): 64–80, reprinted in id., *Keeping the Compound Republic: Essays on American Federalism* (Washington, DC: Brookings Institution Press, 2001.

6. Simon N. Patten, "The Decay of State and Local Governments," *Annals of the American Academy of Political and Social Science* 1 (July 1890): 26–42.

7. Luther Gulick, "Reorganization of the State," *Civil Engineering* 3 (August 1933): 421.

8. Derthick, *Keeping the Compound Republic*, n. 5 above, p. 130.

9. John Gardner, introduction to *The Sometime Governments: A Critical Study of Fifty American Legislatures* (New York: Bantam Books for the Citizens Conference on State Legislatures), p. viii.

10. Alice Rivlin, *Reviving the American Dream: The Economy, the States and the Federal Government* (Washington, DC: Brookings Institution Press, 1992), pp. 86–87.

11. Daniel M. Fox, *The Discovery of Abundance: Simon N. Patten and the Transformation of Social Theory* (Ithaca, NY: Cornell University Press for the American Historical Association, 1967), pp. 13–19.

12. Susan Mettler, "Social Citizens of Separate Sovereignties," in *The New Deal and the Triumph of Liberalism*, ed. Sidney M. Milkis and Jerome M. Mileur (Amherst: University of Massachusetts Press, 2002), p. 243.

13. V. O. Key, *American State Government: An Introduction* (1956; repr., New York: Knopf, 1961), pp. 3–4.

14. Robert H. Wiebe, *Self-Rule: A Cultural History of American Democracy* (Chicago: University of Chicago Press, 1995), pp. 211–62. I thank Edward Berkowitz for help in understanding Wiebe's current reputation among historians.

15. Daniel J. Elazar, *The American Mosaic: The Impact of Space, Time and Culture on American Politics* (Boulder, CO: Westview Press, 1994), pp. 281, 288.

16. Donald F. Kettl, "The Maturing of American Federalism," in *The Costs of Federalism*, ed. R. T. Golembrewsky and A. Wildavsky (New Brunswick, NJ: Transaction Publishers, 1984), pp. 73–88.

17. Donald F. Kettl, *The Transformation of Governance: Public Administration for Twenty-First Century America* (Baltimore: Johns Hopkins University Press, 2002), p. 112.

18. William J. Novak, "The Myth of the 'Weak' American State," *American Historical Review* 113 (June 2008): 752–72.

19. Chung Lae Cho and Deil S. Wright, "Perceptions of Federal Aid Impacts on State Agencies: Patterns, Trends and Variation Across the 20th Century," *Publius* 37, no. 1 (Winter 2007): 103–30.

20. Johnson, *Congress and the New Federalism*, n. 1 above, p. 11.

21. Andrew Karch, *Democratic Laboratories: Policy Diffusion Among American States* (Ann Arbor: University of Michigan Press, 2007).

22. Derthick, *Keeping the Compound Republic*, n. 5 above, pp. 28–29.

23. Ibid., pp. 1–2.

24. William J. Novak, "Public Health Quarantine, Noxious Trades and Medical Policy," in id., *The People's Welfare: Law and Regulation in Nineteenth Century America* (Chapel Hill, NC: University of North Carolina Press, 1996), pp. 191–234, makes similar points, and applies them to states' role in health.

25. Barbara Gutmann Rosenkrantz, *Public Health and the State: Changing Views in Massachusetts, 1842–1936* (Cambridge, MA: Harvard University Press, 1972), p. 1. David A. Moss, *When All Else Fails: Government as the Ultimate Risk Manager* (Cambridge, MA: Harvard University Press, 2002), pp. 92–93, 265–66, documents significant work by state government in reducing, avoiding, and spreading risk in the first half of the nineteenth century.

26. Joseph F. Kett, *The Formation of the American Medical Profession: The Role of Institutions, 1780–1860* (New Haven, CT: Yale University Press, 1968); James C. Mohr, *Doctors and the Law: Medical Jurisprudence in 19th Century America* (New York: Oxford University Press, 1993), esp. "Medical Jurisprudence and the State, 1820–1850," pp. 76–93.

27. Carl F. Ameringer, *State Medical Boards and the Politics of Public Protection* (Baltimore: Johns Hopkins University Press, 1999), pp. 16–17.

28. Johnson, *Congress and the New Federalism*, n. 1 above, passim; Jan Doolittle Wilson, *The Women's Joint Congressional Committee and the Politics of Maternalism, 1920–1930* (Urbana: University of Illinois Press, 2007), is particular useful for the Sheppard-Towner program of grants to the states for maternal and child health.

29. Derthick, *Keeping the Compound Republic*, n. 5 above, pp. 15, 110, 140.

30. Johnson, *Congress and the New Federalism*, n. 1 above, pp. 8, 58.

31. For the Biggs story in this paragraph and those that follow, see Daniel M. Fox, "Social Policy and City Politics: Tuberculosis Reporting in New York, 1889–1900," *Bulletin of the History of Medicine* 49 (Summer 1975): 169–95. Elizabeth S. Clemens argues conversely in *The People's Lobby: Organizational Innovation and the Rise of Interest Group Politics in the United States, 1890–1925* (Chicago: University of Chicago Press, 1997), pp. 319–20. that states' bureaucracies grew at the expense of parties and emphasizes direct links between "state bureaucrats and constituents in which party played little role." Parties mattered, however, in more than a few jurisdictions.

32. Anna E. Rude, "Status of State Bureaus of Child Hygiene," *American Journal of Public Health* 10, no. 10 (October 1920): 772–79. Elizabeth S. Clemons, "Lineages of the Rube Goldberg State: Building and Blurring Public Programs, 1900–1940 in *Rethinking Political Institutions: The Art of the*

State, ed. Ian Shapiro, Stephen Skowronek, and Daniel Galvin (New York: New York University Press, 2006), describes substantial state spending for social welfare and health through charitable organizations, accounting for 25–40 percent of all state spending (p. 198) and calculates that state tax revenues supplied "up to four-fifths" of total spending under federal-state matching programs in the 1920s (p. 203).

33. E. I. Bishop, "Public Health at the Crossroads, *American Journal of Public Health* and *The Nation's Health* 25, no. 11 (November 1935): 1175–80. Nevertheless, the Social Security Act had a significant influence on the work of state health departments. "Prior to the passage of the Social Security Act only five state departments of health had a division for industrial hygiene (i.e. occupational health and safety). By 1938 twenty-five states had established such units," Jennifer Klein observes in *For All These Rights: Business, Labor, and the Shaping of America's Public-Private Welfare State* (Princeton, NY: Princeton University Press, 2003), p. 135.

34. Daniel M. Fox, *Health Policies, Health Politics: The British and American Experience, 1911–1965* (Princeton, NJ: Princeton University Press, 1986), pp. 123–31.

35. Data in this paragraph and the next are from David McKay, *Domestic Policy and Ideology: Presidents and the American State, 1964–1987* (New York: Cambridge University Press, 1989), 28, and Joseph F. Zimmerman, *Contemporary American Federalism: The Growth of National Power* (Westport, CT: Praeger, 1992), p. 117. Leonard D. White concluded that states were "more powerful" in 1950 than in either 1900 or 1920 in *The States and the Nation* (Baton Rouge: Louisiana State University Press, 1953), p. 32.

36. Data in this paragraph and the next are from the National Health Accounts and the author's calculations; the most accessible source of this information is www.cms.hhs.gov/nationalhealthexpendituredata/02 (accessed May 6, 2009).

37. The data and much of the interpretation about higher education and education for the health professions in this section are from Daniel M. Fox, "From Piety to Platitudes to Pork: The Changing Politics of Health Workforce Policy," *Journal of Health Politics Policy and Law* 21, no. 4 (Winter 1996): 825–44; followed by commentaries by five experts and my reply, 845–71. The title is deliberately provocative, and I was surprised when the chief executives of the nation's academic health centers responded enthusiastically to the paper when I gave an earlier version as the keynote of the annual meeting of the Association of Academic Health Centers. After I spoke, the chair of the meeting and of the AAHC board, James Mulvihill (then vice president for Health Sciences at the University of Connecticut) thanked me from the lectern: "You enjoyed giving this talk; and we enjoyed listening to it." I described the Narrator and the Bureaucrat in the Preface to this book; this meeting was their first joint public appearance.

38. *Baker v. Carr*, 369 U.S. 186 (1962); *Reynolds v. Sims*, 377 U.S. 533 (1964).

39. This early description of tension between general and specialized government is in an article and report by Leonard D. White, a founder of the field of public administration: *Scientific Research and State Government*, Reprint and Circular Series of the National Research Council, no. 61 (1925), repr. with additions in *American Political Science Review* 19, no. 1 (February 1925): 38–50.

40. National Association of State Budget Officers [NASBO] and Reforming States Group, *2000–2001 State Health Care Expenditure Report* (New York: Milbank Memorial Fund, 2003).

41. Jonathan Engel, *Doctors and Reformers: Discussion and Debate over Health Policy, 1925–1950* (Columbia: University of South Carolina Press, 2002), p. 302.

42. The use of the word "disingenuously" is descriptive rather than an interpretation, because I was the state official. My colleagues and I hoped that the work would inform decisions about coverage under Medicaid. I tell this story because, breaking the rule I described in Chapter 1, I identify myself as a source for part of it in Daniel M. Fox, *Power and Illness: The Failure and Future of American Health Policy* (Berkeley: University of California Press, 1993), pp. 100, 164.

43. For generic drug laws in the states and Congress, see Dominique A. Tobbell, "Allied against Reform: Pharmaceutical Industry—Academic Physician Relations in the United States, 1945–1970," *Bulletin of the History of Medicine* 82, no. 4 (December 2008): 878–912. I thank Tobbell for directing me to additional sources for this point in the press and a report by the Federal Trade Commission. I do not include citations for many points in this section because most of what I write I learned in conversations, meetings and reading as a public official and a policy adviser since 1965. There are few secondary sources on the subject. Except for anecdotes, I cannot reconstruct what evidence and experience led me to reach the generalizations I offer about the politics of making health policy in the states.

44. The secondary literature on Medicaid understandably focuses on policy and operational details of this vast program. An exception is Sandra Tannenbaum, "Medicaid and Disability: The Unlikely Entitlement," *Milbank Quarterly* 67, suppl. 2, pt. 2 (1989), *Disability Policy: Restoring Socioeconomic Independence*: 288–310.

45. Two useful secondary sources for what follows about Medicaid are Michael Sparer, *Medicaid and the Limits of State Health Reform* (Philadelphia: Temple University Press, 1996), and Paul Castellani, *From Snake Pits to Cash Cows: Politics and Public Institutions in New York* (Albany: State University of New York Press, 1966). Castellani's book is the only scholarly account of Medicaid (that I know of) by a former official who participated in making the policy he describes.

46. Fox, *Health Policies, Health Politics*, n. 34 above, describes the history of regional hierarchies since the early twentieth century.

47. Derthick, *Keeping the Compound Republic*, n. 5. above, pp. 138–52.

48. U.S. Advisory Commission on Intergovernmental Relations, *Regulatory Federalism: Policy, Process, Impact and Reform* (Washington, DC: Government Printing Office, 1984), p. 1.

49. The account of state reform that follows draws on a rich literature, which includes U.S. Advisory Commission on Intergovernmental Relations, *The Question of State Government Capability* (Washington, DC: Government Printing Office, 1985); Richard C. Elling, *Public Management in the States: A Comparative Study of Administrative Reform and Politics* (Westport, CT: Praeger, 1992); Ann O'M. Bowman and Richard C. Kearney, "Dimensions of State Government Capability," *Western Political Quarterly* 41, no. 2 (1998): 341–62; David B. Walker, *The Rebirth of Federalism; Slouching Toward Washington* (Chatham, NJ: Chatham House, 1995; Cynthia J. Bowling and Deil S. Wright, "Public Administration in the United States: A Half-Century Administrative Revolution," *State and Local Government Review* 30, no. 1 (1998): 52–64; and David R. Berman, *Local Government and the States: Autonomy, Politics and Power* (Armonk, NY: M. E. Sharpe, 2003). An article by William Pound, long-serving executive director of the National Conference of State Legislatures, is particularly useful: "Twenty-five Years of Reform," in *Changing Patterns in State Legislative Careers*, ed. Gary F. Moncrieff and Joel A. Thompson (Ann Arbor: University of Michigan Press, 1992), pp. 9–21.

50. On senior state officials' experience of term limits, see *Time Enough? States Respond to Term Limits* (New York: Milbank Memorial Fund and the National Conference of State Legislatures, 1997). These officials reported the support of some business groups for term limits. On the effects of term limits, see *Institutional Change in American Politics: The Case of Term Limits*, ed. Karl F. Kurtz, Bruce Cain, and Richard G. Niemi (Ann Arbor: University of Michigan Press, 2007).

51. Joseph F. Zimmerman, *Congressional Preemption: Regulatory Federalism* (Albany, NY: State University of New York Press, 2005), esp. pp. 7–8.

52. David Benor "Federalism, Pre-Emption, and Obesity Law," 2008 National Summit on Legal Preparedness for Obesity Prevention and Control, June 20, 2008, presents an arresting typology of preemption. Benor has asked me to say that the information in this article does not represent the opinion of his employer, the Office of General Counsel of the U.S. Department of Health and Human Services.

53. David M. O'Brien, "The Rehnquist Court and Federal Preemption: In Search of a Theory," *Publius* 23, no. 3 (Fall 1993): 17.

54. Daniel M. Fox and Daniel C. Schaffer, "Health Policy and ERISA: Interest Groups and Semi-Preemption," *Journal of Health Politics, Policy and Law* 14, no. 2 (Summer 1989): 239–60; William Pierron and Paul Fronstin, "ERISA Pre-Emption: Implications for Health Reform and Coverage" (Issue Brief no. 204, Employee Benefit Research Institute, Washington, DC, February 2008).

55. Henry J. Kaiser Family Foundation, *Employee Health Benefits: 2008 Annual Survey*, § 10, http://ehbs.kff.org/pdf/7790.pdf (accessed April 14, 2009).

56. See *Five States That Could Not Wait: Lessons for Health Reform from Florida. Hawaii, Minnesota, Oregon, and Vermont*, ed. Daniel M. Fox and John K. Iglehart (Bethesda, MD: Milbank Memorial Fund and the People-to-People Health Foundation, 1994; distributed by Blackwell).

57. For a history of the Reforming States Group to 1993, see Kathleen S. Andersen, "The Reforming States Group and the Promotion of Federalism," *Milbank Quarterly* 76, no. 1 (1998): 103–20.

58. Memorandum from Senator Tom Daschle to "Democratic Senators," May 26, 1994 attached to a summary, "State Legislators Talk Health Care Reform." Copy in the files of the Milbank Memorial Fund.

59. "Sure there's frustration. But we've all been through this, and it's not totally unexpected. . . . It's the way democracy works—we're not efficient," Minnesota Democratic State Representative Lee Greenfield told the *New York Times*. See "State Health Officials Strive to Bring the Health Care Debate Home," *New York Times*, September 25, 1994, www.nytimes.com/1994/09/25/us/state-officials-strive-to-bring-the-health-care-debate-home.html?sec=health (accessed April 14, 2009), a guarded account of the negotiations. The Milbank Memorial Fund has the printed Mitchell-Chafee Bill and related documents in its archive at Yale University. This episode is described and contextualized in "Bill Clinton: Kicking the Health Care Can Down the Road," in David Blumenthal and James Morone, *At the Heart of Power* (Berkeley: University of California Press, 2009), pp. 378–81.

60. Reforming States Group, *State Oversight of Integrated Health Systems* (New York: Milbank Memorial Fund, 1997).

61. NASBO and Reforming States Group, *2000–2001 State Health Care Expenditure Report*, n. 40 above.

62. Reforming States Group, "State Initiatives on Prescription Drugs: Creating a More Functional Market," *Health Affairs* 22, no. 4 (July–August 2003): 128–36.

63. See ibid., passim, for quotations in this and the preceding paragraph.

CHAPTER 4

1. Meeting Proceedings, Second Annual Participant Governance Meeting, Drug Effectiveness Project [sic], Center for Evidence-based Policy (CEBP), April 12–14, 2004 (Portland, OR: CEBP), p. 6.

2. For a technical overview of reference drug pricing policy, see Malcolm McClure, "Drug Insurance Utilization Management Policies and 'Reference Pricing,'" *Milbank Quarterly* 83, no. 1 (2005): 131–47. A timely discussion of the applicability of the policy to the United States is Panos Kanavos and Uwe Reinhardt, "Reference Pricing for Drugs: Is It Compatible with U.S. Health Care?" *Health Affairs* 22, no. 3 (May–June 2003): 16–30.

3. Daniel M. Fox and Andrew D. Oxman, "Introduction," in *Informing Judgment: Case Studies of Health Policy and Research in Six Counties* (New York: Milbank Memorial Fund, 2001), www.milbank.org/reports/2001cochrane/010903cochrane.html#introduction (accessed April 7, 2009). The sixth country was South Africa, where policy makers chose to reject research results.

4. Daniel M. Fox, "Evidence of Evidence-Based Health Policy: The Politics of Systematic Reviews in Coverage Decisions," *Health Affairs* 24, no. 1 (January–February, 2005): 114–22.

5. Brook made this statement at a meeting of the Advisory Board, U.S. Cochrane Center, Washington, DC, July 28, 2004.

6. For a summary of states with PDLs by 2004, see Robert Pear and James Dao, "States' Tactics Aim to Reduce Drug Spending," *New York Times*, November 21, 2004, www.nytimes.com/2004/11/21/national/21DRUGS.html (accessed April 7, 2009).

7. Ibid.

8. "Pharmaceutical Preferred Drug Lists (PDLs)—State Medicaid and Beyond," compiled by Richard Cauchi, program director, National Conference of State Legislatures Health Programs. Revised January 3, 2008. Received from Richard Cauchi, June 2008.

9. Meeting Proceedings, First Annual Participant Governance Meeting, [Drug Effectiveness Review Project], Center for Evidence-based Policy (CEBP), October 7–9, 2003 (Portland, OR: CEBP), p. 1.

10. Ibid., p. 7.

11. I base the description of DERP governance and policy in the preceding and following paragraphs on a variety of sources. For the explanation of policy, I rely on Mark Gibson, "When Good Information Truly Matters: Public Sector Decision Makers Acquiring and Using research to Inform Their Decisions," *Journal of Law and Policy* 14, no. 2 (2006): 551–68. In addition, DERP staff made available the minutes of monthly conference calls and annual governance meetings and documents on major policies. Alison Little, the current director of DERP, wrote a useful "DERP History" in February 2008. Pam Curtis (still at CEBP), John Santa (who is now on the staff of Consumers Union), and Marion McDonough (Evidence-Based Practice Center, Oregon Health and Science University) addressed many question in a conference call on March 3, 2008. Mark Gibson reviewed this chapter in draft. The quotations in this section of the chapter are direct quotations from these documents and conversations.

12. Little, "DERP History," n.11, p. 3.

13. DERP, CEBP, "Process for DERP II Topic Prioritization—Revised May 2007."

14. Ibid., p. 2.

15. Little, "DERP History," p. 3.

16. Meeting Proceedings, n. 1 above, p. 10.

17. Fox, "Evidence of Evidence-Based Health Policy," n. 4 above, pp. 117–18; clarified by Mark Gibson in subsequent conversations.

18. Anne McFarlane, then assistant deputy minister of health in British Columbia, at the conference convened by Governor Kitzhaber in Portland, OR, in 2002, described in Chapter 1.

19. Frederick Mosteller, "The Prospect of Data-based Medicine in the Light of ECPC," *Milbank Quarterly* 71, no. 3 (1993): 523–32, esp. p. 531.

20. Joanna Coast, "Is Economic Evaluation in Touch with Society's Health Values?" *BMJ* 329 (November 20, 2004): 1233–36. Similarly, Michael Rawlins, who chairs the National Institute for Health and Clinical Excellence (NICE) in the United Kingdom said in 2008 that the monetary value assigned to a quality-adjusted life year (QALY) is "really a judgment of the economic community": Robert Steinbrook, "Saying No Isn't NICE—The Travails of Britain's National Institute for Health and Clinical Excellence," *New England Journal of Medicine* 359, no. 19 (November 6, 2008): 1977–80.

21. *Valuing Health for Regulatory Cost-Effectiveness Analysis*, ed. L. L. Miller, A. Robinson, and R. S. Lawrence (Washington, DC: National Academies Press, 2006. See also Daniel M. Fox, "The Determinants of Policy for Population Health," *Health Economics, Policy and Law* 1, no. 2 (2006): 401–2, and id., "Values Advocacy and the Politics of Health Policy" (Proceedings of the 13th Annual Policy Conference, Centre for Health Economics and Policy Analysis, McMaster University, May 2000).

22. Alan Williams, an economist who was a major contributor to the development of QALYs, writes that "if you wish to reduce inequalities in people's lifetime experience of health, you have to discriminate against the old" ("Discovering the QALY . . .," in *Personal Histories in Health Research*, ed. Adam Oliver [London: Nuffield Trust, 2005], p. 201).

23. Peter J. Neumann, "Emerging Lessons from the Drug Effectiveness Review Project," *Health Affairs* 25, no. 4 (2006): w268.

24. Alan Maynard, e-mail to Iain Chalmers and Daniel M. Fox, July 25, 2005. Maynard was kinder in a published comment on similar observations I made in 2006, see above, n. 21. A major contribution toward more effective use of economic analysis to inform policy is Gordon H. Guyatt et al., "Incorporating Considerations of Resource Use into Grading Recommendations," *BMJ* 336 (May 24, 2008): 1170–73.

25. David Henry, "Use of Systematic Review / Meta-Analysis in the Australian PBS" (n.d.; e-mail attachment sent by Henry to the author, February 18, 2008).

26. Ruth Lopert to the author, Montreal, July 8, 2008.

27. Bob Nakagawa, e-mail to the author, February 18, 2008.

28. Andrew D. Oxman, e-mail to the author, February 15, 2008, citing M. L. Baum et al., "A Survey of Clinical Trials of Antibiotic Prophylaxis in Colon Surgery: Evidence against Further Use of No-Treatment Controls, *New England Journal of Medicine* 305, no. 14 (October 1, 1981): 795–99. Oxman also called attention to APT Statistical Secretariat, "Collaborative Overview of Randomised Trials of Antiplatelet Therapy," *BMJ* 308 (January 15, 1994): 159–68. Similarly, David Henry brought to my attention E. M. Antman et al.,

"A Comparison of Results of Meta-Analyses of Randomized Control Trials and Recommendations of Clinical Experts: Treatments for Myocardial Infarction," *JAMA* 268, no. 2 (July 8, 1992): 240–48. Iain Chalmers's contribution, by e-mail, to this list of earlier comparative reviews was Iain Chalmers, "Randomized Controlled Trials of Fetal Monitoring 1973–1977," in *Perinatal Medicine,* ed. O. Thalhammer et al. (Stuttgart: Georg Thieme, 1979, 260–65. Chalmers also wrote (February 21, 2008) that he and his colleagues cited other examples of comparative reviews in *Effective Care in Pregnancy and Childbirth,* ed. Iain Chalmers et al. (Oxford: Oxford University Press, 1989.

29. Mark Helfand, e-mail to the author, February 18, 2008.

30. Helfand statement at a meeting of the Advisory Board of the U.S. Cochrane Center with the Steering Group of the Cochrane Collaboration, Providence, RI, March 31, 2005.

31. Marion McDonough to the author, Portland, OR, May 1, 2008.

32. Gibson, "When Good Information Truly Matters," n. 11 above, p. 556.

33. Mark Gibson, e-mail to the author, February 10, 2008.

34. Mark Gibson, "Making the Best Use of Limited Resources for Drug Evaluations" (presentation at Cochrane Collaboration Colloquium, São Paulo, Brazil, October 26, 2007), p. 13.

35. Little, "DERP History," n. 11 above, p. 5.

36. Summary of DERP Governance conference call, September 1, 2005, p. 1.

37. Gibson, "Making the Best Use," n. 35 above, p. 9.

38. The broad outline of the analysis of industry antagonism to DERP in this section emerged during a day-long meeting of Mark Gibson, John Santa, and the author, on August 31, 2006, to assess pertinent documents that had been collected by Santa and other members of the DERP staff. At the time we were considering writing an article on the subject, in part to respond to interest aroused by a talk on the subject by Gibson, "Attacks on Systematic Reviews," U.S. Cochrane Center Conference, Baltimore, July 14, 2006. Following the meeting I extended the analysis. One reason we did not write the article was to avoid being perceived as carrying the battle to the industry rather than responding to its tactics by describing the methodology of systematic reviews in great detail and calling attention to the best available evidence. The generalizations about industry behavior in this section are, therefore, entirely my own; no reader should assume that any member of the staff of DERP or the CEBP or the DERP governance agrees with this analysis. Moreover, at my informants' request, many quotations and statements are unattributed in this section.

39. There is extensive documentation for the statements in this paragraph, as there is for the other paragraphs describing the relationship between the pharmaceutical industry and DERP. A Google search on September 15, 2009, for DERP found 653,008 results, many of which had been generated by the pharmaceutical industry and its surrogates.

40. Mosteller, "Prospect of Data-based Medicine," n. 19 above.

41. The *Cochrane Methods Groups Newsletter*, an annual publication since 1996, reports on advances in and work in progress to improve the methodology of systematic reviews. It will be a fertile source for future historians of science. See www.cochrane.org/newslett/index.htm (accessed April 16, 2009).

42. Quoted in Gibson, "When Good Information Truly Matters," n. 11 above, pp. 560–61.

43. Gibson and Santa in their rejoinder amplified an article they had published several months earlier, replying to a published critique (Neumann, "Emerging Lessons," n. 23 above): Mark Gibson and John Santa, "The Drug Effectiveness Review Project: An Important Step Forward," *Health Affairs* 25 (2006): w272–w275. The same electronic edition of *Health Affairs* also included other articles criticizing and praising DERP.

44. Tom Toolen, "States Misuse Evidence-Based Medicine," *Medical Herald* (New York City), April 2005.

45. Richard Gottfried, e-mail to the author, January 19, 2009.

46. National Association of State Medicaid Directors, *2007 State Perspectives: Medicaid Pharmacy Policies and Practices* (Washington, DC: NASMD, 2007), p. viii.

47. For a review of the legal issues in the case, see Michelle M. Mello, David M. Studdert, and Troyen A. Brennan, "The Pharmaceutical Industry versus Medicaid—Limits on State Initiatives to Control Prescription-Drug Costs," *New England Journal of Medicine* 350, no. 6 (February 5, 2004): 608–13.

48. Daniel M. Fox and Lee Greenfield, "Helping Public Officials Use Research Evaluating Healthcare," *Journal of Law and Policy* 14, no. 2 (2006): 543–45.

49. Ibid., p. 546.

50. An example of the nationwide uptake of the AP article was a story on MSNBC on November 24, 2004, "More States Reviewing Drug Safety Themselves: Joint Project Comparison Shops for Effective Medicine," www.msnbc.msn.com/id/6574759 (accessed April 16, 2009).

51. "Detective Work: Reading Fine Print, Insurers Question Studies of Drugs," *Wall Street Journal*, August 24, 2005, p. A1. For the *New York Times*, see Pear and Dao, "States' Tactics," n. 6 above.

52. Alicia Ault, "Comparison Shop for Pills? A New Tool Lets You. But Experts Say Don't Buy on Price Alone," *Washington Post*, December 21, 2004, p. HE01; Christopher Rowland, "Consumer Reports Turns Focus to Prescription Drugs," *Boston Globe*, December 10, 2004, www.boston.com/business/articles/2004/12/10/consumer_reports_turns_focus_to_prescription_drugs?pg=2 (accessed April 16, 2009).

53. Alan Murray, "Political Capital: Trade Group's Fight against Drug Review is Self-Defeating," *Wall Street Journal*, November 30, 2004, p. A4.

54. Rich Daly, "U.S. Unique in Approach to Funding Prescription Plans," *Psychiatric News* 41, no. 14 (July 21, 2006): 1, http://pn.psychiatryonline.org/cgi/content/full/41/14/1-a (accessed April 16, 2009).

55. Ezekiel Emanuel and Ron Wyden, "A New Federal-State Partnership in Health Care: Real Power for States," *JAMA* 300, no. 16 (October 22–29, 2008): 1931–34. See also Ezekiel J. Emanuel, Victor R. Fuchs, and Alan M. Garber, "Essential Elements of a Technology and Outcomes Assessment Initiative," *JAMA* 298, no. 11 (September 19, 2007): 1323–25.

56. Statement of Gail Shearer, Testimony before the Subcommittee on Health of the House Committee on Ways and Means, June 12, 2007, www .waysandmeans.house.gov/hearings.asp?formmode=view&id=6112 (accessed April 8, 2009).

57. Daniel M. Hartung, Kathy L. Ketchum, and Dean G. Haxby, "An Evaluation of Oregon's Evidence-Based Practitioner-Managed Prescription Drug Plan," *Health Affairs* 25, no. 5 (2006): 1423–32. Two other studies evaluated DERP's process but do not include data on its effectiveness: Ryan Padrez, Tanisha Carino, Jonathan Blum, and Dan Mendelson, *The Use of Oregon's Evidence-Based Reviews for Medicaid Pharmacy Policies: Experience in Four States* (Menlo Park, CA: Henry J. Kaiser Family Foundation, 2005); and David Bergman, Jack Hadley, Neva Kaye, Jeffrey Crowley, and Martha Hostetter, *Using Clinical Evidence to Manage Pharmacy Benefit: Experience in Six States* (New York: Commonwealth Fund, 2006).

58. Author's calculations from data provided by members of the DERP Governance using data on total Medicaid spending by state from the database maintained by the Henry J. Kaiser Family Foundation, www.statehealthfacts .org (accessed April 8, 2009).

59. John Santa in conference call with the author, March 11, 2008.

60. These data are public, in slides prepared for a talk by an official of Idaho Medicaid: Tami Eide, "Newer Anticonvulsants: Managing On and Off Label Use" (American Drug Utilization Review Society, February 28, 2008).

61. Peter Cunningham, "Medicaid Cost Containment and Access to Prescription Drugs," *Health Affairs* 24, no. 3 (2005): 780–89.

CHAPTER 5

1. Jonathan Lomas, "The In-Between World of Knowledge Brokering," *BMJ* 334 (January 20, 2007): 130.

2. A superbly crafted example of research that assesses knowledge transfer from the point of view of organizations that sponsor research is John N. Lavis, Dave Robertson, Jennifer M. Woodside, Christopher B. McCleod, and Julia Abelson, "How Can Research Organizations More Effectively Transfer Research Knowledge to Decisionmakers," *Milbank Quarterly* 81, no.2 (June 2003): 221–48. For an example of research that takes account of some of the work of making policy, see Christopher J. Jewell and Lisa A. Bero, " 'Developing Good Taste in Evidence: Facilitators and Hindrances to Evidence-Informed Health Policymaking in State Government," *Milbank Quarterly* 86 (June 2008): 177–208. The authors thank Lee Greenfield, a policymaker in Minnesota,

some of whose work I describe elsewhere in this book, for comments on the article in draft.

3. John N. Lavis, Suzanne E. Ross, Gregory L. Stoddart, Joanne M. Hohenadel, Christopher B. McLeod, and Robert G. Evans, "Do Canadian Civil Servants Care about the Health of Populations?" *American Journal of Public Health* 93, no. 4 (2003): 658–63.

4. John N. Lavis, Suzanne E. Ross, Jeremiah E. Hurley, et al., "Examining the Role of Health Services Research in Public Policymaking," *Milbank Quarterly* 80, no. 1 (March 2002): 125–54.

5. Craig Mitton, Carol E. Adair, Emily McKenzie, Scott B. Patten, and Brenda Waye Perry, "Knowledge Transfer and Exchange: Review and Synthesis of the Literature," *Milbank Quarterly* 85, no. 4 (December 2007): 729–68.

6. Steven Lewis, "Toward a General Theory of Indifference to Research-Based Evidence," *Journal of Health Services Research and Policy* 12, no. 3 (July 2007): 166.

7. Fitzhugh Mullan, Ellen Ficklen, and Kyra Rubin, *Narrative Matters: The Power of the Personal Essay in Health Policy* (Baltimore: Johns Hopkins University Press, 2006), p. 2.

8. The most comprehensive account of the broadening of methodology is in the annual volumes of the *Cochrane Methods Groups Newsletter* (see Chapter 4, n. 41) For a different approach to methodology that focuses on evaluating change in health care processes, see *Knowledge to Action: Evidence—Based Health Care in Context,* ed. Sue Dopson and Louise Fitzgerald (Oxford: Oxford University Press, 2005). Also see Stephen G. West et al., "Alternatives to the Randomized Controlled Trial," *American Journal of Public Health* 98, no. 8 (August 2008): 1359–66.

9. U.S. Congress, Office of Technology Assessment, *The Impact of Randomized Clinical Trials on Health Policy and Medical Practice: Background Paper,* OTA-BP-H-22 (Washington, DC: Office of Technology Assessment, 1983), http://govinfo.library.unt.edu/ota/Ota_4/DATA/1983/8310.PDF (accessed April 16, 2009).

10. *Effective Care in Pregnancy and Childbirth,* ed. Iain Chalmers, Murray W. Enkin, and Mark J. Keirse, 2 vols. (Oxford: Oxford University Press, 1989).

11. Iain Chalmers describes and documents the scarcity of both systematic reviews and primary studies in an editorial introducing a "series of articles on areas of practice where clear and robust evidence is lacking": "Confronting Therapeutic Ignorance: Tackling Uncertainties about the Effects of Treatments Will Help to Protect Patients," *BMJ* 337 (August 2, 2008): 246–47.

12. For the National Institutes of Health mission statement, see www.nih.gov/about/index.html#mission (accessed April 16, 2009).

13. Imogen Evans, Hazel Thornton, and Iain Chalmers, *Testing Treatments: Better Research for Better Healthcare* (London: British Library, 2006), p. 99.

This book is a trenchant introduction to the issues discussed in this section. It is available without charge at www.jameslindlibrary.org/testing-treatments .html (accessed April 16, 2009).

14. Mike Clarke, Sally Hopewell, and Iain Chalmers, "Reports of Clinical Trials Should Begin and End with Up-to-Date Systematic Reviews of Other Relevant Evidence: A Status Report," *Journal of the Royal Society of Medicine* 100 (2007): 187–90.

15. Richard A. Rettig, Peter D. Jacobson, Cynthia M. Farquhar, and Wade M. Aubry, *False Hope: Bone Marrow Transplantation for Breast Cancer* (New York: Oxford University Press, 2007). Moreover, as discussed in Chapter 2 of this book, the persuasiveness of the technology assessments (TA) of this and other interventions was limited because most of the organizations that did TA in the United States had been forced by the politics of health services into a business model that required proprietary publication rather than publication in peer-reviewed scientific journals. Of course politics can trump science even when convergence seems to have occurred. In a state that had a formal process for assessing new technology when the issue of mandating ABMT surfaced, legislators set it aside when the wife of the Speaker of the House wanted the treatment.

16. Because this book focuses on politics and policy I have not presented technical details about methodology of systematic reviews. For readers who want some detail, a useful introduction is Evans et al., *Testing Treatments,* n. 13 above. For those who want even more technical detail, succinctly presented, a good source is Khalid S. Khan, Regina Kunz, Jos Kleijnen, and Gerd Antes, *Systematic Reviews to Support Evidence-based Medicine: How to Review and Apply Findings of Healthcare Research* (London: Royal Society of Medicine Press, 2003).

17. *Milbank Quarterly* 71, no. 3 (September 1993): 345–48, 411, 532.

18. Lee Greenfield, Sheldon H. Greenfield, Paul D. Cleary, and B. D. Colen, *Evaluating the Quality of Health Care: What Research Offers Decision Makers* (New York: Milbank Memorial Fund, 1996).

19. Sean Tunis and Steven D. Pearson, "Coverage Options for Promising Technologies: Medicare's 'Coverage With Evidence Development," *Health Affairs* 25, no. 5 (2006): 1218–30.

20. Peter R. Orszag, director, Congressional Budget Office, "Research on the Comparative Effectiveness of Medical Treatments: Options for an Expanded Federal Role," Testimony before the Subcommittee on Health, Committee on Ways and Means, U.S. House of Representatives, June 12, 2007, www.cbo .gov/doc.cfm?index=8209 (accessed April 16, 2009).

21. For documentation of scientific, clinical and policy issues in comparative effectiveness research, see www.iom.edu/cms/28312/RT-EBM. aspx (accessed April 16, 2009).

22. *Knowing What Works in Health Care: A Roadmap for the Nation,* ed. Jill Eden, Ben Wheatley, Barbara McNeil, and Harold Sox (Washington, DC: National Academies Press, 2008).

23. The American Recovery and Reinvestment Act of 2008. H.R. 1, http://frwebgate.access.gpo.gov-bin/getdoc.cgi?dbmar=111_cong_bills& docid=f:hlenr.pdf (accessed May 8. 2009); Robert Steinbrook, "Health Care and the American Recovery and Reinvestment Act," *NEJM* 360, no. 11 (March 12, 2009: 1057–60.

24. Ceci Conolly, "Comparison Shopping for Medicine: Obama's Stimulus Package Funds Research on Cutting Costs," *Washington Post*, March 17, 2009, A2, www.washingtonpst.com/wp-dyn/content/article/2009/03/16/AR2009031602913.ht.ml (accessed May 9, 2009); Barry Meier, "A New Effort Reopens a Medical Minefield," New York Times, May 7, 2009, B2, www.nytimes.com/2009/05/07/business/07compare.html (accessed May 8, 2009).

25. Because I am not aware of any research on the subject of this and subsequent paragraphs on research careers, I rely on what I have seen, heard and read as an official of public agencies, universities, and a foundation, and as a participant in research on health services and policy.

26. Victor M. Montori and Gordon H. Guyatt, "Progress in Evidence-Based Medicine," *JAMA* 300, no. 15 (October 15, 2008): 1874–76. This article describes the uptake of evidence-based medicine since publication of a seminal article on this "new paradigm of medical practice," Evidence-Based Medicine Working Group, "Evidence-Based Medicine: A New Approach to Teaching the Practice of Medicine," *JAMA* 268, no. 17 (November 4, 1992): 2420–25.

27. Niteesh K. Choudhry, Robert H. Fletcher, and Stephen B. Soumerai, "Systematic Review: The Relationship between Clinical Experience and Quality of Health Care," *Annals of Internal Medicine* 142, no. 4 (2005): 260–73.

28. David Pryor, "Quality Transformation at Ascension Health: The Role of Transparent Reporting" (presentation to a conference convened by the Saskatchewan Health Quality Council, Saskatoon, June 27, 2008). I have benefited from conversations on the subject of this paragraph over several years with Pryor, David Lawrence, Robert Crane, Murray Ross, and Paul Wallace of Kaiser Permanente, Gordon Hunt of Sutter Health, and Woodrow Myers, formerly of Wellpoint.

29. James Thompson, telephone conversation, May 15, 2008 and e-mail exchanges with the author on April 17 and May 12, 2008.

30. David E. Kindig et al., *Value Purchasers and Health Care: Seven Case Studies* (New York: Milbank Memorial Fund, 2001).

31. Robert S. Galvin and Suzanne Delbanco, "Why Employers Need to Rethink How They Buy Health Care," *Health Affairs* 24, no. 6 (2005): 1549–53.

32. Robert Galvin and Suzanne Delbanco, "Between a Rock and a Hard Place: Understanding the Employer Mind-Set," *Health Affairs* 25, no. 6 (2006): 1548–55.

33. Mark Gibson and John Santa, "Designing Benefits with Evidence in Mind," Issue Brief no. 290, Employee Benefit Research Institute, February

2006; e-mail exchange between Paul Fronstin and the author, February 29 and March 3, 2008.

34. Robert S. Galvin, "Still in the Game—Harnessing Employer Inventiveness in U.S. Health Care Reform," *New England Journal of Medicine* 359, no. 14 (October 2, 2008): 1421–23.

35. E. A. McGlynn, S. M. Asch, J. Adams, J. Keesey, J. Hicks, A. DeCristofaro, E. R. Kerr, "The Quality of Health Care Delivered to Adults in the United States," *New England Journal of Medicine* 348, no. 26 (June 26, 2003): 2635–45.

36. Jessie Gruman, e-mail to the author, January 26, 2009.

37. Ray Moynihan demonstrates his expertise in many publications and films; see, e.g., *Evaluating Health Services: A Reporter Covers the Science of Research Synthesis* (New York: Milbank Memorial Fund, 2004).

38. Stephanie Saul, "Test of Drug for Diabetes in Jeopardy," *New York Times*, May 22, 2007, www.nytimes.com/2007/05/26/business/26drug.html; "Ignoring the Warnings, Again?" ibid., May 25, 2007, www.nytimes .com/2007/05/25/opinion/25fri1.html?pagewanted=print (both accessed April 16, 2009). An e-mail message from Jeffrey Lerner of ECRI Institute alerted me to Saul's story while I was in Scotland. I then sent an e-mail to another medical writer for the *New York Times*, with whom I have worked for several decades, complaining that no single RCT is as powerful as a state-of-the-art systematic review. He replied that my claim about systematic reviews was news to him. The editorial appeared several days later.

39. Gail Shearer, Consumers Union, e-mail, with attachments, to the author, March 25–26, 2008.

40. Martiga Lohn, "Web Sites to Help Consumers Save on Drugs," Associated Press, June 22, 2006, http://wcco.com/health/web.site.website .2.372708.html (accessed May 6, 2009).

41. For this paragraph and the next, Gail Shearer, n. 39 above; and supplementary e-mail to the author, May 31, 2008.

42. Roger Dobson, "UK Doctors Show Most Interest in Falls Among Elderly People, But French More Curious about Type 2 Diabetes," *BMJ* 336 (April 12, 2008): 797; for information about free access to the Cochrane Library, see www3.interscience.wiley.com/cgi-bin/ mrwhome/106568753/AccessCochraneLibrary.html (accessed April 16, 2009).

43. Peter C. Gøtzcshe, "Believability of Relative Risk and Odds Ratios in Abstracts: Cross Sectional Study," *BMJ* 333 (July 19, 2006): 231–34; Gøtzcshe and colleagues also documented that Cochrane reviews are more credible than reviews supported by the pharmaceutical industry and other organizations: Anders W. Jorgensen, Jørgen Hilden, and Peter C. Gøtzcshe , "Cochrane Reviews Compared with Industry-Supported Meta-Analyses and Other Meta-Analyses of the Same Drugs: Systematic Review," *BMJ* 333 (October 6, 2006): 782–85.

44. Gardiner Harris, "Psychiatrists Top List in Drug Maker Gifts," *New York Times*, June 27, 2007, A14, www.nytimes.com/2007/06/27/health/psychology/27doctors.html (accessed April 16, 2009).

45. Jana Kolarik Anderson et al., *Vendor-Healthcare Professional Gift-Giving, Marketing and Compliance*: American Health Lawyers Association, December 12, 2007, updated June 2008, www.Compliance-institute.org/pastCIs/2008/Conference/700s/711/AHLA-WhitePaperVendor-HCP-GiftGiving.pdf (accessed May 8, 2009); Robert Steinbrook, "Disclosure of Industry Payments to Physicians," *New England Journal of Medicine* 359 (August 7, 2008): 559–61; Scott Allen, "Leaders Nip, Tuck Healthcare Policy: Limits Enacted on Drug Firm Gifts," *Boston Globe*, August 11, 2008, www.boston.com/news/local/articles/2008/08/11/leaders_nip_tuck_healthcare_policy (accessed April 16, 2009); Barry Meier, "An Rx for Ethics: New Rules on Doctors and Medical Firms Amid Conflict Concerns," *New York Times*, January 24, 2009, B1.

46. Kim Dixon, "Senate Revises Drugmaker Gift Bill," Reuters, May 13, 2008, www.reuters.com/article/politicsNews/idUSN1340711320080513 (accessed April 16, 2009).

47. Troyen A. Brennan, et al. [eleven authors], "Health Industry Practices That Create Conflicts of Interest: A Policy Proposal for Academic Medical Centers, *JAMA* 295, no. 4 (January 25, 2006): 429–33.

48. AAMC-AAU Advisory Committee on Financial Conflicts of Interest in Human Subjects Research, *Protecting Patients, Preserving Integrity, Advancing Health: Accelerating the Implementation of COI Policies in Human Subjects Research* (Washington, DC: Association of American Medical Colleges, 2008).

49. Toby Manthey, "Medicaid Rx Program Saves $20 million; Critics Assert State System Doesn't Prescribe the Best for Every Patient," *Arkansas Democrat-Gazette*, December 9, 2006.

50. "As Drug Costs Continue to Rise State Legislatures Become Increasingly Proactive" (electronic press release), Research and Markets, Dublin, Ireland, June 28, 2007, not available on the company's Web site in September 2008), but see www.redorbit.com/news/health/984094/as_drug_costs_continue_to_rise_state_legislatures_become_increasingly/index.html (accessed May 31, 2009).

51. Bob Nakagawa, British Columbia Ministry of Health Services assistant deputy minister for pharmaceutical services, and members of his staff gathered the Canadian data at my request. A recent systematic review of studies of detailing found that "alone or when combined with other interventions [it has] effects on prescribing that are relatively consistent and small, but potentially important": M. A. O'Brien et al., "Educational Outreach Visits: Effects on Professional Practice and HealthCare Outcomes," *Cochrane Database of Systematic Reviews*, no. 4 (October 17, 2007), http://mrw.interscience.wiley.com/cochrane/clsysrev/articles/CD000409/frame.html (accessed April 17, 2009).

52. For a similar argument, see Peter D. Jacobson, "Transforming Clinical Practice Guidelines Into Legislative Mandates: Proceed with Abundant Caution," *JAMA* 299 (February 28, 2008): 208–10. More broadly, Pascal Lehoux writes that "an increased circulation of evidence-based knowledge about technology can be effective in improving the regulation of health technology only if it is accompanied by transparent deliberative processes"; *The Problem of Health Technology: Policy Implications for Modern Health Care Systems* (New York: Routledge, 2006), pp. xxi, 187–91.

53. Nicole M. Bellows, Helen Ann Halpin, and Sara B. McMenamin, "State Mandated Benefit Review Laws," *Health Services Research* 41, no. 3, pt. 2 (June 2006): 1104–23, identify twenty-six states with these laws and document the wide range in research methods among states. I have been unable to locate the source the authors cite, but a citation in a 2009 paper I reviewed claimed that thirty states had mandated benefit review laws in 2007.

54. For a history of the program, see Maryland Health Care Commission, *Annual Mandated Health Insurance Services Evaluation*, January 19, 2006, http://mhcc.maryland.gov/health_insurance/annualmandaterpt.2008.pdf (accessed May 8, 2009).

55. John Colmers, e-mail to the author, September 3, 2008.

56. Mark Gibson. e-mail to the author, August 19, 2008.

57. Richard Cauthi, Pharmaceutical Preferred Drug Lists (PDLs)—State Medicaid and Beyond, National Conference of State Legislatures, Health Program, Revised January 3, 2008; See Chapter 1, note 1.

58. Washington State Representative Eileen Cody, "Evidence Based Practice in Washington State" Presentation at the Public Health Law Conference, Centers for Disease Control and Prevention, Atlanta, GA, June 2006; updated for a panel on "U.S. State-Based and International Programs," Conference on How Effective Is Value-Based Purchasing in the Public and Private Sectors?, Washington DC, December 2, 2008.

59. Kansas Administrative Regulation 30–5–58, July 6, 2001.

60. Nialson Lee, e-mail, with attachments, to the author, March 24, 2008.

61. Sara Singer, Linda Bertthold, et al. [nine authors], *Decreasing Variation in Medical Necessity Decision Making* (Center for Health Policy, Stanford University, for the California Health Care Foundation, August 1999); e-mail correspondence, Linda Bergthold, Sara Singer, and the author, March–April, 2008. Mark D. Smith, president of the California Health Care Foundation, facilitated these exchanges. Despite what Bergthold and Singer recall, the most extensive discussion of evidence in the report (p. 39) merely says that "a coverage decision may be based on evidence-based practices" and that "coverage policies . . . may include evidence of effectiveness."

62. J. Hutton, P. Trueman, and C. Henshall, "Coverage with Evidence Development: An Examination of Conceptual and Policy Issues," *International Journal of Technology Assessment in Health Care* 23, no. 4 (2007): 425–35. However, at a panel at the annual meeting of Health Technology Assessment International, in Montreal (July 8, 2008), Jean Slutsky, a senior official of

AHRQ in the United States, noted that there is "no systematic process for determining the best opportunities for conditional reimbursement." For a survey of programs in western European countries that use the best available evidence to inform decisions about medical necessity, see Bernhard Gibis, Pedro W. Koch-Wulkan, and Jan Bultman, "Shifting Criteria for Benefit Decisions in Social Health Insurance Decisions," in *Social Health Insurance Systems in Western Europe,* ed. Richard B. Saltman, Reinhard Busse, and Josep Figueras (Maidenhead, Berkshire, UK: Open University Press, 2004), 189–206.

63. Twenty-three of the twenty-six states that require hospitals to report adverse events also require them to analyze their root causes using one of several validated methodologies for reviewing evidence of system failure; Jill Rosenthal and Mary Tacach, *2007 Guide to State Adverse Event Reporting Systems,* State Health Policy Survey Report (Washington, DC: National Academy for State Health Policy, 2007).

64. The DQA is Section 515 of the Consolidated Appropriations Act of 2001 (PL, 106–554). A trenchant critique of its implementation is Chris Mooney, *The Republican War on Science* (New York: Basic Books, 2005). A more recent investigation of the difficulty of establishing processes through which the best available evidence can inform policy in the environmental field is Mark Bowen, *Censoring Science: Inside the Political Attack on Dr. James Hansen and the Truth of Global Warming* (New York: Dutton, 2008). Thomas McGarity and Wendy Wagner, *Bending Science: How Special Interests Corrupt Public Health Research* (Cambridge, MA: Harvard University Press, 2008), array considerable detail about how corporate advocates and their political allies (at times including regulators) have discredited or suppressed research on potential health hazards, especially from environmental toxins.

65. See www.ucsusa.org/scientific_integrity/abuses_of_science/a-to-z-guide-to-political.html (accessed April 10, 2009).

66. Evan Doran and David Alexander Henry, "Australian Pharmaceutical Policy: Price Control, Equity, and Drug Innovation in Australia," *Journal of Public Health Policy* 29 (2008): 106–20. For other evidence of manufacturers' recent efforts to change Australian policy, and to use the argument about innovation to do so, see Andrew Searles, Susannah Jeffreys, Evan Doran, and David A. Henry, "Reference Pricing, Generic Drugs and Proposed Changes to the Pharmaceutical Benefits Scheme, *MJA* 187, no. 4 (August 20, 2007): 236–39. My source for the behavior of the present Australian Labor Party government prefers to remain anonymous.

67. Julie-Anne Davies, "P[harmacy] B[enefit] S[cheme] Foots Bill for Kids' Prozac," *The Australian,* July 23, 2008. www.theaustralian.news.com.au/story/0,25197,24063150–23289,00.html (accessed April 17, 2009).

68. Merrill Goozner, "State Medicaid Programs Threatened by Free Trade Deals?" Gooznews.com, January 24, 2009, www.gooznews.com/archives/001310.html, citing www.wcl.american.edu/pijip/go/blog01222009 (both accessed April 10, 2009).

Index

AAMC (Association of American Medical Colleges), 33, 48, 68, 129

Abel-Smith, Brian, 30

ABMT (Autologous Bone Marrow Transplantation), 112, 153n15

academic health centers (AHCs), 35–37, 40–41, 63–64, 66–68, 69

academics, and research on health services, viii, 34–35

access to health care, under Medicaid, 12–13, 66, 93–94, 97

advisers, to policymakers, vii, 2, 29, 89, 112, 129, 158n64

Advocate, narrative voice of, 136n28

Aetna Health Insurance, 118

Agency for Health Care Policy and Research (AHCPR), 47–49, 80

Agency for Healthcare Research and Quality (AHRQ), 8, 49, 84–85, 90–91, 100, 113, 115

AHCPR (Agency for Health Care Policy and Research), 47–49, 80

AHCs (academic health centers), 35–37, 40–41, 63–64, 66–68, 69

AHRQ (Agency for Healthcare Research and Quality), 8, 49, 84–85, 90–91, 100, 113, 115

alternative health reform bill of 1994, 73–74, 146n59

AMA (American Medical Association), 23, 24, 26, 33, 38, 65, 119

American Board of Internal Medicine Foundation, 124

American Hospital Association, 27, 33

American Medical Association (AMA), 23, 24, 26, 33, 38, 65, 119

American Recovery and Reinvestment Act of 2009 (ARRA), 104, 111

Anderson, Odin, 35, 136–37n36

Annenberg Foundation, 121

Anthem Health Insurance, 118

Arnstein, Sherry, 45

ARRA (American Recovery and Reinvestment Act of 2009), 104, 111

Ascension Health, 118

Association of American Medical Colleges (AAMC), 33, 48, 68, 124, 129

Australia: convergence and, 78, 130; independent research and, 130; pharmaceutical industry and, 78, 79, 130; physicians' autonomy and, 130; public access to Cochrane Collaboration systematic reviews and, 123; RCTs and, 7; researchers who inform policymaking for health and, 116; RSG and, 4; systematic reviews of pharmaceutical drugs and, 87, 111; TA and, 46

Text:	10/13 Aldus
Display:	Aldus
Compositor:	Toppan Best-set Premedia Limited
Indexer:	Naomi Linzer
Printer & binder:	Maple-Vail Book Manufacturing Group